Dr. Generic
Will See You Now

Oscar London / Carlota Cohen
arlen
Cohen
Cohn

848-1933

By the same author
Kill As Few Patients As Possible
Take One As Needed

Dr. Generic Will See You Now

33 Rules for Surviving Managed Care

Oscar London, M.D., W.B.D.

Ten Speed Press
Berkeley, California

Some chapters of this book originally appeared in *The Washington Post* and *San Francisco Focus Magazine*.

Ten Speed Press
P.O. Box 7123
Berkeley, California 94707

Distributed in Australia by E.J. Dwyer Pty. Ltd., in Canada by Publishers Group West, in New Zealand by Tandem Press, in South Africa by Real books, and in the United Kingdom and Europe by Airlift Books.

Cover and text design by Fifth Street Design
Cover illustration by Akiko Shurtleff

Library of Congress Cataloging-in-Publication Data
on file with the publisher.

Printed in Canada

First printing, 1996

1 2 3 4 5 6 7 8 9 20 – 00 99 98 97 96

To Joan, Jenny, Ted, Diane, Sydney, and Haley

CONTENTS

INTRODUCTION:

Welcome to Managed Care

What the Public Health Doctor fails to prevent, the Private Doctor tries to cure; what the Private Doctor fails to cure, the Specialist tries to improve; what the Specialist fails to improve, the Mortician beautifies.
—Anonymous

This just in—we're all going to die. Getting there, of course, is half the fun. It should be *all* the fun, but life, especially in this century, has become a killjoy. Until recent years, American medicine had greatly enhanced our ability to reach three score and ten in reasonably good shape and in pretty good humor. Then along came Managed Care, and the prospect of an untimely death suddenly became, if not attractive, certainly cost-effective.

Welcome to Managed Care—health care managed by business school Ph.D.'s to save bucks and fill their coffers, rather than by medical school M.D.'s to save lives and heal their coughers.

In the good old days of 1993 when your doctor still practiced fee-for-service medicine, he worked as his own boss, not a de facto employee of a health insurance company. Your doctor could readily order any test or drug to improve your health or save your life and, if necessary, send you off to any specialist without a hassle (but with a hefty fee).

Admittedly, fee-for-service was costly up front, but the comprehensive care of yore could often save you $100,000 in hospitalization bills, plus eternal convalescence from an otherwise preventable illness. For Americans, old-fashioned comprehensive care was simply the best medicine practiced in the world and, I have to concede, the most expensive.

Under fee-for-service, your doctor was paid according to how many patients he saw and how many tests he ordered. Then in 1994 Managed Care exploded. Now your doctor is paid a fixed sum per patient per year, whether or not he sees the patient or orders any tests.

With fee-for-service, a number of doctors charged astronomic fees for such dramatic procedures as coronary bypass surgery, cataract operations, and hip replacements, when merely substantial fees would have been appropriate. These superstar doctors and their five-star hospitals helped kill the goose that had laid their golden eggs for decades. The fat goose has now been replaced by a skinny chicken called Managed Care.

That skinny chicken is running free over the whole range of American medicine and, instead of the chicken, patients and their doctors are now in the soup. What that skinny chicken has been laying in the laps of doctors is not in any way, shape, or form a golden egg. As a patient, you'd better save up your own nest egg to shell out for a coronary bypass at age 83, when your Care Managers inform you that you're too old to qualify.

Through immensely popular Health Maintenance Organizations (HMOs), Managed Care is rapidly taking over American medicine. (In my book, "Managed Care" and "HMO" are synonymous.) Millions of unsuspecting patients have signed up for HMOs, enticed by low premiums and the promise of comprehensive care. The low premiums are real—the promise of comprehensive care is science fiction.

In 1994, the seven biggest for-profit HMOs used a greedy 17.3 to 27.1 percent of their revenues from premiums for administrative costs and profits (compared to just 4 percent of the premiums for administrative costs reported by not-for-profit Kaiser Permanente). They also awarded cash and stock options to their CEOs that averaged 7 million dollars each, and focused their strategic planning on quarterly profits and low payments for direct medical care.

It is not rare for a single HMO to have accumulated billions of dollars in profits just in the past few years. Some medical economists believe these galactic profits translate into significant losses for patients and doctors.

As always, you get what you pay for: bargain-basement premiums buy you bargain-basement medicine. Welcome to Managed Care. Your employer has negotiated to get you into a cheap HMO that may require you to change doctors and *will* require you to change health habits.

To survive Managed Care, you must learn to take care of yourself. The utter necessity to take charge of your own life before entrusting it to a doctor is the great contribution of Managed Care. Before you're forced to see a doctor in the purgatory of his office or the hell hole of the emergency room, read the 33 rules I have compiled to help you survive Managed Care. I offer you a bracing tonic of common sense, laced with a dollop of nonsense. Sip it while I savage what's bad about Managed Care, and try to salvage what's good.

To help you survive Managed Care, your doctor needs your assistance. Like God, whom doctors unsuccessfully have tried to emulate for eons, your physician can best help those who help themselves.

NOTE: In referring to a doctor, I will often use the pronoun, "his," rather than "his or her," owing to my own gender and, with a bow to Managed Care, for the sake of economy.

RULE 1:

Don't Let an HMO Give You Nickel-and-Dime Care for Your Million-Dollar Body

As my colleague, Gerald the proctologist, sees it, "Fee-for-service did too much for the patient. Managed Care is doing too little." Of course, Gerald can be faulted for seeing things from a rather narrow point of view (or, as he puts it, "through a glass darkly").

Managed Care has corrected some of the abuses of fee-for-service, which included outrageous duplication of expensive equipment, such as a five-million-dollar MRI unit in every hospital in town when only one MRI could have amply served the community. Did the hospitals encourage excessive use of this high-profit, high-tech diagnostic tool? Does a radiologist drive a BMW?

Under fee-for-service, a hospital profited according to how many beds were filled and how many tests were ordered. Its administrators did not frown upon lengthy hospitalizations and costly procedures. Under Managed Care, the HMO pays each hospital a lump sum whether or not its beds are filled. The hospital's expenses are carved out of this lump and what's left over, if anything, is profit.

Thus, profits to the hospital diminish whenever a bed is occupied or an X-ray taken and increase with each bed kept empty and each X-ray not ordered. Hospitals are now discouraging admissions, lengthy hospital stays, and complex procedures. Many hospitals under Managed Care are now half-empty, as are the pockets of their administrators.

More and more hospital cases are being treated in outpatient day-care centers and sent home the same day. As a result, home nursing programs have markedly improved under Managed Care while hospital nursing programs have slipped badly. In some cases, desperately strapped hospitals are replacing costly registered nurses with much cheaper, marginally trained "Nurse Assistants." The lesson to the patient: stay out of hospitals, and flush that pack of cigarettes down the toilet. (According to each of the reports of the U.S. Surgeon General produced since 1964, cigarette smoking is the single most important source of preventable disease and premature death.)

Your old friend the doctor has become your new enemy, the gatekeeper, and the sign on the gate says, "Keep Out." To see an expensive specialist, you must pass through more doors than a visitor to San Quentin.

These days, your doctors are told by Managed Care, "Keep it cheap or get out of my insurance company!" Under severe budgetary constraints (which also include a huge drop in physician income), your doctors are prevented from recommending certain drugs, tests, and specialists, calculated as too expensive by Managed Care. When this happens, patient care suffers while Managed Care thrives.

The budgetary cuts of Managed Care will likely discourage the invention of life-saving (but expensive) high-tech equipment and state-of-the-art drugs, which have defined the excellence of American medicine. Eventually, when the best and brightest of college undergraduates get word of the hassle of doctoring under Managed Care and the free-fall of doctors' incomes, they will change their academic pursuits from pre-med to pre-flight. (In contrast to a doctor under Managed Care, the captain of a Boeing 747 is not required to pilot his ship from a seat in economy class and earns an average of $280,000 per year.)

With Managed Care, a high school graduate, using a software program in a distant office, informs your doctor that the tests he ordered for you cannot be done because their cost-benefit ratio is too high. That is, the cost to the insurance company is deemed too high compared to your benefit. I will readily admit to ordering tests that, in retrospect, did not benefit many patients. But those same costly tests can also help cure a few patients who might be inadequately diagnosed under the squeeze of Managed Care. In one year of a medical practice, these seven or eight great cases are what separate a good doctor from a mediocre one.

Until it loosens its purse strings, Managed Care is threatening the good doctor with extinction. By the lights of Managed Care, a good doctor is one who orders as few tests and medications for his patients as possible. To wit, the good doctor of Managed Care is beginning to resemble the mediocre doctor of fee-for-service.

The great doctor of Managed Care, of course, is the patient herself who stays lean and well-exercised, doesn't smoke, drinks little or no alcohol, unfailingly wears her seat belt, and has ancestors who lived into their 90s. (A male patient seldom outlives a female patient and remains the weaker sex under Managed Care.)

An alarmingly popular form of Managed Care is called "capitation," wherein the insurance company pays the doctors and hospitals a fixed, flat fee for each patient whether the patient is treated or not. Under capitation, doctors are often given a bonus for ordering fewer tests on their patients and sending them to fewer specialists than in the old days.

Under fee-for-service, doctors were rewarded for seeing as many patients as possible. Under capitation, they are rewarded for seeing as few patients as possible; ergo, your doctor will be happy not to see you. Seemingly overnight, fee-for-service doctors have changed into flee-from-service doctors. Welcome to Managed Care.

With gold-rush fever, Medicare patients are swarming into capitation plans that promise zero premiums. Zero premiums result from Medicare, who with your permission has sold your aging body to the lowest bidder—your HMO. Zero premiums are also made possible by the slashing of your doctor's income to a relatively small fee each year for your simply being enrolled in his practice. To stay economically alive, your doctor must sign up hordes of patients, who will eventually, by the sheer weight of their numbers and their reasonable demands, drive him to an early grave. The tombstone will be marked: The Doctor Is In. Have a Seat.

You might well ask why we doctors have contracted with these proliferating, profiteering HMOs. It's because most of our patients have joined these HMOs, lured by the half-kept promise of low premiums and comprehensive care. Thus, your doctor is given the choice of sitting in an empty office and going broke instantly or running through a crowded office and going broke eventually. The doctor who refuses to be capitated becomes, in effect, decapitated—a Managed Care chicken with its head cut off.

Our secretaries are also somewhat less than euphoric under Managed Care. Have you noticed that their former friendliness is beginning to wear a bit thin? Not only do they have to assist us clinically, but must also fill out countless forms and be put on telephone hold for eternities in order to persuade your HMO to permit you to see a specialist.

Good grief! The American medical specialists used to be the envy of the world, not just for their handsome incomes, but mostly for their superb clinical skills. With all due respect to my colleagues in internal medicine and family practice, we can't give you first-class care without easy access to specialists.

It's in the best economic interests of your HMO to sign up as many of you as possible—while you're still reasonably healthy. Managed Care is marvelous for your health if you don't get sick. Many HMOs admirably sponsor preventive services, such as anti-smoking clinics, AA groups, weight loss programs, and exercise clubs.

But wait until you get older and, necessarily, sicker. You may find yourself no longer the darling of your HMO, which is happy to collect your premiums but not your grievances. Heaven forbid you should get really sick, as we all will someday. Let's say you somehow survive and need prolonged home care with expensive equipment and drugs. In the time of your final need, how long will your HMO support your costly care until it decides to cut you dead? Figuratively speaking.

The cost-consciousness of Managed Care is the fertile soil in which the government's health reforms will eventually take root. One of these days, the 41 million formerly uninsured Americans will join Managed Care. These are people who were not robust enough to qualify for private health insurance or rich enough to afford the pre-miums. They will be swept into the waiting rooms of overworked and underpaid doctors where, with luck, they'll receive the same mediocre care you are presently being told you are enjoying.

Gerald the proctologist refuses to encourage his kids to go to medical school, "because I don't want them to accuse me of child abuse eight years later." Despite the burdens of Managed Care, I myself concur with another colleague's remarks to an entering class of medical students: "Some will tell you that the profession is underrated, unhonored, under-paid, its members social drudges—the very last profession they would recommend to a young person. I would rather tell you of a profession honorable above all others, one which, while calling for the highest pow-ers of the mind, brings you into such warm personal contact with your fellow man that the heart and sympathies of the coldest nature must need be enlarged thereby." This was from the address of Sir William

Osler, the greatest internist of all time, to the entering class at McGill University in 1877.

How can you as a patient get optimal care under Managed Care? Good question. Have a seat. Doctor London will be able to examine your form just as soon as you complete your portion.

If you want to be covered by your fair share of a threadbare, overstretched blanket of health care, you will have to become a tosser and a turner, a grabber and a shover, a mover and a shaker—all aerobically sound activities that will ensure you prompt care, if you need it, from a traditionally good doctor. You have to insist loudly and clearly on seeing the doctor, whether he wants to see you or not. You must demand to see a specialist when your heart says you must and your doctor says you can't.

In the final analysis, what will save you, as well as Managed Care, is a healthy dose of self-care and self-promotion.

Patient, heal thyself.

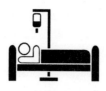

RULE 2:

Your Doctor Is Your Humble Servant—His Secretary, Your Imperial Highness

A doctor is nothing more than your servant. Humbly and in some cases grumbly, he is at your service. If you treat your doctor with the respect you would tender a kind and wise butler, he will anticipate your every need, make your life more comfortable, and be at your beck and call at all hours.

On the other hand, your doctor's secretary is the Queen. It behooves you to get on her good side. After all, she wields the absolute power to make appointments for you on the spur of the moment. If you are to be ruled by a good queen instead of an evil one, regard her with the deference and affection a British subject would confer on any member of the Royal Family (with the exceptions of Charles, Diana, and Fergie).

As your Queen, the secretary is empowered to command your HMO to let you see any specialist you desire, let you have exotic drugs not "on the formulary," and, if you bow low enough, bestow on you the restroom key. Hail the doctor's protectress and yours, his secretary!

As your lowly servant, I'm astonished by how many of you treat my secretary as a commoner and me as royalty. You've got it backwards! I'm trained and required to be nice to you no matter how you behave. My secretary operates under no such constraints. In any disagreement before her throne, I always take the side of my Queen. Otherwise, she'd keep me locked in the Tower of London, as I call my office, and throw away the key.

Try being imperious with Her Highness, my most-exalted secretary, and she will banish you to the darkest corner of my waiting room and keep you there filling out forms till night falls. Be rude to my secretary and your pharmacist will suddenly not have your prescription ready and ask you, his old friend, how you spell your last name.

Fail to smile at my secretary and turn your charm instead on me and, before you know it, you will find yourself dressed in a paper gown three sizes too small and locked in a tiny exam room with moldering periodicals whose best articles have been ripped out. While you cool your bare heels on the cold linoleum, your humble servant will be waiting on patients who came after you but were able to cajole the Queen with flattery and boxes of soft-centered chocolates.

Remember Her Serene Majesty on her birthday! Lay fresh produce and warm breads at her feet! Gasp in delight at her snapshots of her children, the Prince and Princess! Compliment her on the faithfulness of her copy machine, the succinctness of her faxes, the telephonic tact with which she puts you on hold! Hail the doctor's secretary from whom all good health flows, as well as the juiciest gossip!

Meanwhile, I look forward to serving you. If it pleases the Queen.

RULE 3:

If You Don't Wear Condoms because They Dull Sensation, Dying Young Will Dull Sensation Even More

Managed Care would save itself a bundle if it distributed condoms as freely as it does newsletters.

While having sex, more teenage boys wear sneakers than condoms. For the world's favorite indoor sport, why more Nikes than Trojans? Safe socks? No, the modern, high-tech sneaker is considered sexier than the laceless, graceless condom.

Managed Care should urge makers of condoms to take a cue from the sports shoe CEOs: Add pressure-activated colored lights. Attach lateral stabilizing straps for a snug fit. Install dual inflatable airbags. Get endorsements from basketball stars.

The fact that every male teenager in America is guaranteed a pair of Nikes under the Constitution tends to bolster the sneaker market. If the teenager's parents refuse to buy him a pair, he can plead cruel and unusual punishment (Amendment VII). If his parents can't afford to buy him a pair, he can exercise his right to bear arms (Amendment II), and rob a convenience store (Amendments VII-XI) to get the necessary cash. In contrast to the $100 pair of Nikes which teenage boys have been known to kill for, you can't give Trojans away.

My solution is to appeal to every teenage boy's darkest secret—his wish to become President someday. What teenage boy has seen Bill Clinton jogging on TV without lusting to fill his sneakers? (Though all viewers agree the presidential shorts should have been left in the briefing room.) The medium is the message: The President not only has all the Nikes he wants (missiles as well as sneakers), but he has a gang of Secret Service agents to run with him so no one can steal them!

Mounting a TV advertising blitz, I'd remind every teenage boy (and girl, while I'm at it) that you can't become President if you don't use condoms. I'd remind them that George Washington, the father of our country, never had children of his own because whenever Martha and George played post office (an intimate game invented by Benjamin Franklin), she made sure they used a "French letter." According to his wife's diary, Martin van Buren customarily wore three condoms at once! To quote a White House confidante, Teddy Roosevelt "never cried 'Charge!' in his bedroom until he had put on his cavalry hat and his condom."

To glorify safe sex, I urge manufacturers of condoms to choose brand names that evoke presidential role models. For example, give high schoolers a choice of Tricky Dick, Slick Willie, or Bedtime for Bonzo.

RULE 4:

Manage Your Own Care

Okay, here goes. This is the drill you must follow to survive Managed Care. Your doctor will no longer call you to do these things. You call him or her.

Unless members of the middle class (same initials as Managed Care) pay for a few essentials out of pocket, they are in danger of having mediocre medicine practiced on them. Those who receive the best medicine are the lower class and the upper class. Members of the lower class visit the emergency room as you would visit your doctor's office. By and large, the ER treats them well and by law can't evict them. For their own care, the upper class (e.g., the CEOs of HMOs) fly first class to the Mayo Clinic (same initials as Managed Care, but with a different attitude toward specialists).

A Hepatitis B vaccination costs $150 for a series of three shots. Your HMO won't pay for it. Stick it to them for not sticking it to you, then pay for it yourself. It's an extremely safe and effective vaccine. Hepatitis B is transmitted the same way as AIDS, but is much easier to catch, can make you as sick, and kill you as dead.

Get a diphtheria-tetanus shot every ten years. Starting at age 50, get a flu shot every year. At age 65, get a pneumonia shot once.

One baby aspirin daily definitely helps prevent heart attacks and strokes and may help prevent esophageal and colon cancer.

Have a general physical exam once by age 30, twice during your 40s, three times during your 50s and yearly after 60.

At age 30, ask your doctor to order the following tests: CBC, Chem 20, LDL and HDL cholesterol, TSH, and urinalysis. First, your doctor will be impressed at your medical sophistication; second, he'll catch hell from your HMO for ordering so many tests; third, you'll be able to learn from the test results if you're suffering in silence from a variety of preventable or treatable ailments, such as anemia, diabetes, kidney disease, coronary heart disease, hepatitis, and thyroid trouble. If you pass these tests and continue to feel well, you can wait until 40 to have them repeated. If you fail one or more of these tests, you might not make it to 40 if you ignore your doctor's advice.

Women, examine your breasts monthly, have a doctor examine them every six months, and get a mammogram yearly after 50. Start at 40 if your mother or sister had breast cancer. Have Pap smears annually till you have three normal ones in a row, then repeat every few years.

If your mother or sister had ovarian cancer, get an annual, trans-vaginal, pelvic sonogram after age 40, even if you have to pay for it yourself.

Starting at age 50, submit to a colonoscopy, sigmoidoscopy, or barium enema every five years, unless you've never cheated on your income tax, in which case the IRS will exempt you from colon cancer.

Men over 50: Get a rectal exam each year by a doctor with a slim, tapered index finger to check for prostate cancer. If you'd rather die of aggravation than prostate cancer, get an annual PSA (prostate specific antigen) and hope it's negative, because if it's positive, it may or may not signal prostate cancer. This uncertainty sets you on the road to terminal aggravation where your doctor, who has been there since the advent of Managed Care, will meet you halfway.

Since hypertension is the high road to a stroke, have your blood pressure checked yearly. Seeing a doctor is a major cause of high blood pressure, otherwise known as white-coat or office hypertension. Either measure your blood pressure yourself in the discomfort of your own home or choose a doctor, like me, who wears a navy-blue blazer.

If the upper number is above 140 and the lower number above 90, start blood pressure pills right away, then change your lifestyle. Lose the weight, lower the salt, and increase the exercise until you look and feel like a million bucks. If you tend to put on weight mostly in the abdomen, losing 15 to 30 pounds and keeping it off might cure your hypertension. Then you can try going off the pills. Don't be surprised if your blood pressure shoots back up. At least when you resume your Zestril, you'll still look and feel like a million bucks, which is about what a stroke costs in hospitalization, rehabilitation, grief, and lost income.

Check your skin for brown moles that have turned black, red, white, or blue—those changing spots could be the makings of a melanoma, the most unforgiving of all cancers. Avoid intense sunburn or chronic suntan. Too much sunlight is hell's own fire—if it doesn't kill you with melanoma, it will destroy your beauty with wrinkling and eat away at your scalp, nose, and arms with less aggressive cancers known as basal and squamous cell carcinomas. Start wearing sun block in childhood and you'll have the skin of a teenager at 50. If you women doubt me, compare your skin above your bra line with that below. The trouble is, almost all of us receive over 95 percent of our lifetime sun exposure by age 22.

Floss daily unless you put your teeth in a glass of water at night, in which case, floss weekly (as penance for not flossing until it was too late).

If you feel down on yourself, unaccountably weary and weepy, if you wake up several hours after drifting off and can't get back to sleep, if you have a headache or backache that has defeated two or more doctors, if you're starting to see the bright side of suicide, and if nothing amuses you (not even this book), you might want to bring up the subject of Prozac with your doctor. Since the advent of Managed Care, he's probably been taking it himself.

Become a shrieking smoke alarm if you detect a cigarette in the mouth of your spouse or child. If you yourself smoke, don't scatter your ashes on the living room carpet lest you give your family an idea of how and where to dispose of your remains. (Comparative government statistics: annual deaths from tobacco—400 thousand; alcohol—100 thousand; firearms—35 thousand.)

Two drinks a day for men, one for women, or none for all. One reason the average IQ of college students in America is that of a three-year-old macaque is that over half of our undergrads are immersing their brains in lager instead of logic. It's a good thing these sloshed kids are getting a college education; when they're 40, they'll need the superior income that a B.A. commands to pay for their stay in the Betty Ford Clinic. For too many, B.A. stands for bachelor of alcoholism. Too many of the best and brightest are graduating *magna cum loaded*.

At the end of your life, your family will miss you more if you die from smoking than from drinking. Cigarettes merely rot your lungs; alcohol rots your soul. By the time you die from too much booze, your family can't wait for you to go. It takes a long time for a stiff to become a stiff. Resentment sets in long before rigor mortis does. The dirty secret about alcohol is that it raises one's HDL or good cholesterol. This means that as many as 300 thousand Frenchmen die each year of cirrhosis with wide-open coronaries.

Sleep deprivation is a national epidemic and causes an insidious drain on the quality of your everyday life. If you're logging less than eight hours of shut-eye and are tired most of the day, add at least 45 minutes to your sleep time by hitting the sack earlier or grabbing an afternoon nap. You might meditate, as I do, 15 minutes, twice daily. (My early-evening "meditation" tends to slide into a comatose and rejuvenating nap; thus, my efforts to raise my consciousness often render me unconscious. For more on meditation, see Rule 24.)

Finally, to defer calling 911 indefinitely, diet to the point of looking good for your body type—and exercise. Become a stranger to Taco Bell, a galley slave to your rowing machine, an Edmund Hillary to your Stairmaster, a ski-bum to your NordicTrack. Or—see if I care—enjoy 20 minutes of aerobic sex three times a week while watching Jane Fonda's first workout tape, *Barbarella*.

RULE 5:

Appoint Me Surgeon General for a Day

Surgeon General Oscar London's Orders of the Day

1. All HMOs must request Surgeon General's approval before denying a patient access to any test, drug, or specialist deemed necessary by his or her primary care physician. In the spirit of Managed Care, all such requests to this office from HMOs will be thoughtfully rejected.
2. Check every man, woman, and monkey for HIV. Results available on demand to would-be sex partners and other organ grinders.
3. To insure nation-wide immunizations, no child will be admitted to Disneyland or Disneyworld without reporting to Shot Land just outside main gate. Doctors dressed as Doc give shots while Snow White nurses dry blood, sweat, and tears. After work, a booster shot of Wild Turkey for each Snow White and Doc.
4. Legalize cocaine, heroin, marijuana, gambling, and prostitution. Build post office annexes to house government casinos, crack houses, and bordellos. These facilities will be staffed by U.S. Post Office employees to discourage patronage. (For example, "I'm sorry, sir, prostitution is window three—you're in the keno line.") Civil service tradition of lying down on job selectively tolerated.
5. With trillions of dollars saved from order number four, saturate prime-time TV with infomercials on horrors of cocaine, heroin, gambling, prostitution, alcohol, and cigarettes. If that doesn't work, let's party.
6. Sentence tobacco company CEOs to execution by firing squads made up of lung cancer patients. Requests by CEOs for final ciga-

rette denied on grounds of second-hand smoke hazard to firing squad.

7. Instruct Justice Department to permit sale of semi-automatic rifles only to card-carrying members of NRA who obtain notes from a urologist certifying erectile dysfunction. That is to say, sale of Uzis permitted to members in good standing.

RULE 6:

Take Two Aspirin and Call Me in the Millennium

Of the three men in the room, one was bored, one was anxious, and one was dead. The 64-year-old pathologist, heavy-set and bald, languidly prepared to make his incision. I was the anxious one—an intern, age 23, my face stubbled with a three-day growth of beard, my eyes fixed intently on the pathologist's scalpel blade.

On the metal table lay the suntanned body of the male patient, age 43. Staring up at me with dilated pupils, he was a handsome man, with a lean, well-muscled body, a clean-shaven face, and a full head of brown, impeccably groomed hair. From the standpoint of general appearance, the patient seemed the least likely of the three men in the room to have died.

On a sultry summer afternoon in 1962, we were gathered in the chilly morgue of the Jewish Hospital of St. Louis to perform an autopsy. I was apprehensive at the prospect of assisting at an autopsy, my first, even though it promised to be that euphemism for something unpleasant: "a learning experience."

It was not as if I had never seen a dead body before—it was that I had never seen one looking so unmarked by disease or injury. What most distressed me was the patient's beautiful head of hair—and what was about to be done to it. Its careful grooming revealed not only the patient's vanity, painfully touching under the circumstances, but the confidence of a man, not yet 50, who assumed he would live forever—or at least until his next haircut.

The patient had been brought in D.O.A. at noon from the YMHA handball courts. The cause of his sudden death could have been a stroke, a heart attack—or anything. Grumbling about the necessity of examining the brain of the stricken athlete, the pathologist casually began scalping him. It was an artful incision within the hairline, allowing the mortician, who would pick up the remains later, the opportunity to showcase the body in such a way as to elicit the obligatory comment, "He looks so natural." (As if a man in a business suit lying in a casket could ever be perceived as looking natural.)

After sawing out a bone flap in the skull, the pathologist handed me the brain to weigh. I had received my Doctor of Medicine degree a few months before, but I did not become a physician until this moment. Unwittingly, the jaded pathologist was teaching me clinical detachment, an acquired trait that must somehow be reconciled by physicians with their inborn qualities of fear and empathy.

Hamlet held up a skull and said, "Alas! poor Yorick. I knew him, Horatio; a fellow of infinite jest, of most excellent fancy; he hath borne me on his back a thousand times, and now, how abhorred in my imagination it is!" Hamlet, in other words, was not clinically detached.

Wearing rubber gloves that were a size too large for me, I tremulously rested the patient's brain on a small scale. With a strained voice that would not have carried to the first row of the Globe Theater, I announced, "1,450 grams." The most important thing I learned was not how much the brain before me weighed, but, with the simple act of weighing it, how well I could disguise my reeling thoughts.

Looking for signs of a stroke, the pathologist began cutting the brain into thin slices. At length, he glanced up at me and said the Yiddish word for nothing: "Gornischt."

He then straightened up, sighed, and cleaved the patient with a perfectly straight, 24-inch incision from the base of the neck to the pubic bone. At that moment I would have killed for a cigarette. Five minutes later, as the pathologist cut through the patient's lungs, I gave up smoking forever. They were tar-blackened and bloated from 25 years of chain-smoking. But it wasn't lung disease that killed him.

By the time the pathologist had me weigh the heart, I had lost my anxiety. I was now totally absorbed in his methodical quest for the exact cause of death. In the patient's left coronary artery he found it.

"Look," he said, prodding with the tip of his scalpel blade the purple belly of the tiny killer.

He had deftly sliced the major branches of the patient's coronary arteries into fine segments. They were full of cheesy deposits of fat, a joint contribution of the dairy and tobacco industries. But the yellowish globs clogging the man's arteries were only accessories to his demise. His assassin was a purple blood clot, the size of a match head, that choked off his fat-narrowed left coronary artery.

In the 1960s, it was assumed that a blood clot was the hit man in a heart attack. Then, for two decades, the clot so often found lurking at the scene of the crime was downgraded to an innocent bystander— a postmortem coagulation. Surveillance was lifted from a major suspect in the deaths of millions of people. It has taken another 15 years, and scores of clinical papers, to re-affirm—at least for the time being—that the sudden jelling of blood in a fat-choked artery delivers the *coup de gráce*.

Now we take small doses of aspirin to prevent that fatal event and are given large doses of clot-dissolving drugs to treat an acute myocardial infarction. Will an aspirin a day keep the pathologist away?

I emerged from that morgue, a newborn physician, 33 years ago. I have spent the intervening decades trying to keep myself from being wheeled back in.

Regrettably, in the past 10 years there has been a notable drop in the number of autopsies performed in the United States. The malpractice threat may have something to do with doctors' reluctance to recommend postmortem exams to bereaved families. Doctors are thus missing an opportunity to learn from their mistakes before burying them and family members are being deprived of clinical information on inheritable diseases, knowledge of which might delay their own funerals.

For more than three decades since my first autopsy, I have exhorted my patients to eat chicken and fish, to exercise, and to quit smoking. Lately, I've prescribed Pravachol for those whose LDL cholesterols are elevated. If I have helped some of my patients forestall their heart attacks, they can thank that well-groomed man of 43, lying on his back in the morgue, staring up at me.

He would have been only 76 now.

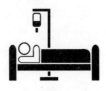

RULE 7:

Only Fatheads Don't Count Calories

Pity the makers of junk food! These bloated merchants of suet are now required to reveal the calorie count of every item they package. What a boon this is to Managed Care—more information means more profit from less disease. This formerly secret information, now appearing in boldface type, will put the moguls of grease on skid row. At night these purveyors of fat thrash about in their king-sized beds like harpooned whales.

I can envision an emergency board meeting of the Slippery Pig Crackling Company. The Chairman slumps at the head of the oiled walnut table, his pale, porcine face buried in his fat, pink hands.

CHAIRMAN: *(moans)* 8000 calories! We can't print that!

WEATHERBEE (marketing): We have to, boss. Our six-ounce bag of Slippery Pig Cracklings actually contains 8,389 calories, but the FDA will let us round it off to the nearest thousand.

CHAIRMAN: 8000 calories! The only customers who'll buy our product will be members of the Hemlock Society!

SCHUMAKER (advertising): Nah, boss, our little plastic bags would never fit over their heads. What we might do is declare each of the 14 cracklings in our six-ounce bag "one serving" and—let's see *(fingers dance over pocket calculator and tongue goes 'tuh-tuh-tuh')*—that comes to only 480 calories per serving! Can you live with that, boss?

CHAIRMAN: No, and neither can our customers. How can we sleep nights pushing a product that causes premature heart attacks? *(He lights up a cigarette.)* Hell, what is a goddamn calorie anyway?

SEMMELWEISS (research and development): It's the measurement of heat energy in food required to raise the temperature of one gram of water one degree centigrade.

CHAIRMAN: Heat energy? So when we eat cracklings, why don't we get hot instead of fat?

SEMMELWEISS: Just had an idea, boss. Let me borrow your lighter. Watch this—lean back everybody! (*He ignites plastic bag of Slippery Pig Cracklings. A huge ball of fire shoots up to ceiling, falls, and burns through oiled walnut table. The overhead sprinklers turn on, dousing fire and drenching board members.*) That's it! I've just invented the first bag of Slippery Pig Fire Starter!

SCHUMACKER: (*thrilled*) Right on, Semmelweiss! Our slogan'll be, "Nothin' Like a Cracklin' Fire!" What d'ya say, boss? Think we can change the labels in time for Christmas?

CHAIRMAN: (*enigmatically*) No, that won't be necessary. Well, I guess the fat's in the fire—meeting adjourned.

The following Sunday at three in the morning, the Slippery Pig Crackling factory in Merwin, Alabama caught fire. It burned to a crisp in a blaze that took firefighters eight days to control and insurance investigators 30 seconds to conclude that something about the great Slippery Pig Crackling fire was not entirely kosher.

RULE 8:

For Her 50th Birthday, Give Your Spouse a Two-Carat Diamond and a Five-Foot Colonoscopy

Q. What's worse than lying down and allowing someone to pass five feet of tubing slowly through the entire length of your colon?
A. Colon cancer.

Piously citing cost-benefit ratios, Managed Care doesn't believe everyone should have a colonoscopy after age 50. Instead, they recommend the less extensive and cheaper sigmoidoscopy. As soon as the young CEOs of Managed Care turn 50 themselves, guess what they'll demand from one of their captive doctors? That's right—a colonoscopy. When I turned 50, I begged my friend Gerald the proctologist to use the long tube on me rather than the short one. Our phone conversation went as follows:

GERALD: Oscar, I'd be happy to do a colonoscopy on you. What are your symptoms?

OSCAR: I'm scared and I'm 50.

GERALD: Your HMO won't let me inflict a colonoscopy on you just because you're a nervous old wreck. Has anybody in your immediate family had colon cancer?

OSCAR: Nope.

GERALD: Polyps?

OSCAR: Nope.

GERALD: Have you had a change in bowel habits or lost weight?

OSCAR: Nope.

GERALD: For God's sake, Oscar, you're not giving me any criteria for doing a colonoscopy! Have you ever had rectal bleeding?

OSCAR: Nope. I just have a 50-year-old colon and I don't want to wait for a polyp up there to turn into cancer.

GERALD: Come on, Oscar, just a little streak of blood? Think back—you've got to give me criteria. Otherwise, I won't colonoscope you, even out of professional courtesy.

OSCAR: Why not?

GERALD: Because a colonoscopy is a very discourteous thing to do to a human being, let alone a friend and colleague. Even the American Cancer Society promotes sigmoidoscopy for screening.

OSCAR: But a sigmoidoscope lets you see only the left half of my colon. What if I have a polyp in the right half? What does the American Cancer Society say to that?

GERALD: "All donations are tax deductible." Oscar, tell me you saw one drop of blood and I'll do a colonoscopy.

OSCAR: Well, a few years back I thought I saw a little blood, but then I remembered we ate beets the night before.

GERALD: But it could have been blood?

OSCAR: Yeah, but it was the beets—who knows?—maybe it was blood.

GERALD: Get your tush over here at seven tomorrow morning.

So Gerald had his HMO-approved indication and I had my colonoscopy. It revealed a pre-malignant polyp, the size of a small beet, in the lining of the right side of my colon. My punishment for telling a little white lie was the opportunity to bare my London derrière and have a large black tube worried through my colon. With a snare, Gerald quickly removed what he saw in the light at the end of my tunnel and saved my life.

Thanks to the use of intravenous sedatives and narcotics during the colonoscopy in Gerald's cubbyhole, I dozed through most of the procedure. I was thus spared the additional agony of being a captive audience while Gerald harangued at length on the issue of prayer in public schools. (By the way, there are no atheists in cubbyholes in a proctologist's office.)

Like lung cancer, the tragedy of colon cancer is that by the time you feel the symptoms, it's usually grown too large or spread too far to be cured.

The trick is to zap a benign polyp before it turns into a cancer six to ten years later. You can't zap a polyp growing in the right side of the colon, as mine did, through a two-and-a-half-foot-long sigmoidoscope that reaches no farther than the left half of the colon. You need a colonoscope to go the whole nine yards. In the last several years, increasing numbers of premalignant polyps have been discovered lurking in the right half of the colon, out of reach of the sigmoidoscope, which, according to Gerald, is "a half-assed colonoscope."

There is no good way to prevent and cure colon cancer without a timely colonoscopy. If your stool specimen shows no sign of blood, if your family is free of colon cancer, if you have no intestinal symptoms, you will be hard pressed to find a doctor willing to perform a colonoscopy on you just because you've turned 50. Your friendly neighborhood proctologist would be happy to sigmoidoscope you at 50, but unless your symptoms scream colon polyps or cancer he will not touch you with a ten-foot pole, let alone a five-foot colonoscope.

Tell your doctor it wasn't the beets—anything—to qualify you for a colonoscopy. If you or your proctologist insist, get a sigmoidoscopy and see if I care. Wait! Better than a sigmoidoscopy and probably as revealing as a colonoscopy is an air-contrast barium enema. See if you can persuade your primary-care doctor to order this uncomfortable but revealing X-ray. Then, if the barium enema shows a polyp on the right side of the colon, you receive the bonus of a colonoscopy to remove it. You're welcome.

The sticker price of an Olympus colonoscope with all the bells and whistles is just over $12,000—about what you'd pay for a pretty good used minivan. That's what a colonoscopy feels like—a pretty good used minivan inching the wrong way down a one-way street called your colon.

A colonoscopy costs about a thousand bucks and, according to Managed Care, the yield of polyps is too small to justify that expense for everyone over 50. A $200 sigmoidoscopy is what they'll try to sell you. After all, as the comfortably colonoscoped CEOs of Managed Care aver, only 5 percent of the population at large dies of colon cancer. But I say if it's your cancer, then 100 percent of your population of one dies. When you realize that carcinoma of the colon is the second most common cancer, maybe you should offer to pay for your colonoscopy out of pocket.

Better yet is my friend Gerald the proctologist's modest proposal to erect Colonoscopy Luxury Highrises—privately owned, government-subsidized centers devoted solely to routine colonoscopies. He envisions a cylindrical skyscraper (designed to resemble the Olympus colonoscope) rising in each state of the union. For example, soaring 80 stories above the Nevada desert, Rump Towers of Las Vegas would be filled with sound-proofed, air-conditioned cubbyholes through which cocktail waitresses would pass, dispensing laxatives and keno cards.

As Gerald plans it, whenever one of Rump Towers' proctologists (dressed in a long white coat with sequined lapels) chances upon a polyp during the course of a colonoscopy, bells will start ringing inside the customer's rectum. Suddenly, a show girl will dash into the room and dump 100 shiny silver dollars into the doctor's lap. After all, you don't want an unhappy proctologist doing your colonoscopy, do you?

If Seeing Your Old Friend Makes You Depressed, Your Old Friend Is Depressed

Before they commit suicide, few patients call their doctor to complain about feeling depressed. Usually depressed patients call for help when they develop the *physical* symptoms of depression, such as chronic backache, headache, and fatigue. The treatment of depression has been revolutionized by Prozac; the diagnosis of depression is still in the Dark Ages. Managed Care would rather pay for your Prozac than for your psychiatrist; they figure that, like a picture, one Prozac is worth a thousand words.

Major depression seems to be related to low concentrations in nerve tissue of serotonin, a brain hormone that acts like Tanqueray gin. Unfortunately, the only way to measure serotonin concentrations is to ask patients for a bit of their brain tissue. To date, patients have been largely unwilling to give their doctors a piece of their mind.

Often depression is apparent to your family and friends before it is to you, and they may be shy about confronting you with this unpleasant observation. You may be so used to being depressed that you don't know you're suffering from it. Listen to your family and friends. They are being made miserable by your moodiness and may be your last hope for getting relief before you kill yourself or remain sad the rest of your life.

In the event you've driven off your family and friends, here's a checklist for the diagnosis of major depression. If you have five or more of these nine symptoms and at least one of the first two, call your doctor—you are in serious, but eminently treatable, trouble:

1. Depressed mood most of the day, nearly every day. Depression may be subjective or objective (depression observed, even though you deny being depressed).
2. Markedly diminished interest or pleasure in all, or almost all, activities (anhedonia).
3. Significant weight gain or loss. Weight loss is more common; only 20 percent of depressed patients gain weight.
4. Insomnia or excessive sleep. The classic symptom of early-morning awakening is almost specific for major depression; about 20 percent of depressives would like to sleep all day.
5. Either excessive restlessness or inactivity.
6. Chronic fatigue or low energy. (The much maligned Epstein-Barr virus has been blamed for these symptoms, which often disappear with Prozac.)
7. Feelings of worthlessness or excessive guilt.
8. Diminished ability to think or concentrate, or indecisiveness.
9. Recurrent thoughts of suicide or death.

People bent on committing suicide often drop clues to family and friends, who spend the rest of their lives scoured with guilt for not having recognized these subtle, fatal hints. One clue is a sudden cheerfulness in a chronically sad person—this improved mood can result from the relief afforded by a final decision to kill oneself. Other distant warnings involve repeated, joking reference to death and dying and to funerals. Any marked change in behavior—dropping out of work or school, greatly increased consumption of alcohol or other drugs—that lasts for more than two weeks should alert family and friends to bring in a psychiatrist. Especially among teenagers, a sudden giving away of valued possessions can be a harbinger of suicide.

A dangerous time for seriously depressed patients is the first two to three weeks after starting an anti-depressant pill. Some suicide-bent patients are literally too immobilized by their depression to summon the energy to carry it off. In the first few weeks after being started, an anti-depressant can provide this lethal energy before it removes the suicidal urge.

After I moved to Berkeley in the spring of 1965 to begin my medical career, it didn't take me long to find a depressed patient. I found the unhappiest man I ever met at home, but it was not during a house call.

He answered the door of his old, brown-shingled home only after I rapped the brass knocker three times in rapid succession. My previous single, diffident tap had been met with silence. What was I doing knocking on a stranger's door in Berkeley, shortly after 3:00 P.M. on a Sunday afternoon?

I was newly arrived in the San Francisco Bay Area from the Midwest and had approached the house with a tourist's arrogance. What had occasioned my intrusion was the sight of a huge, magnificent rhododendron bush in the front yard. Standing over six feet tall, it was festooned with scores of blood-red blossoms the size of party balloons. God, what a sight!

You have to be from the Midwest to appreciate my awed delight at the profusion of enormous and glorious flowers blooming everywhere I looked in the Bay Area. In the harsh climate of St. Louis, we dearly earn our few skimpy blossoms; in the Bay Area, they blithely give away the flower shop. My wife and I had recently bought a house in El Cerrito, just north of Berkeley, and were in the midst of a landscaping frenzy.

When I drove past the rhododendron in front of the old Berkeley house on Spruce Street, I slammed on my brakes as if the crimson bush were a stop light. At that moment, the most important thing in my life was to learn the name of this vivid specimen so I could own one of my own.

On opening his door, the owner of the rather seedy house seemed disinclined to share my enthusiasm. He was a pale, thin, bearded man in his late 50s. He was dressed in a dingy, white T-shirt, khaki shorts, and sandals. His sunken, dull-brown eyes did not precisely light up at the sight of a tall, overfed young man in a Glen plaid, three-piece suit whose clean-shaven face was dimpled in a most ingratiating smile.

In fact, the sullen man who stood before me looked for all the world as if he had been interrupted during an elaborately planned suicide. If he had not been interrupted during one, his appearance indicated that he would certainly initiate one as soon as he could get rid of me.

"Excuse me, sir," I said. "But I couldn't help admiring your rhododendron. Do you happen to know its name, by any chance?"

He stared at me for several seconds, then wordlessly closed the door in my imploring face.

Undeterred, I drove over to Berkeley Horticultural Nursery and spotted a newborn version of the very specimen growing in a gallon can. The pleasant owner informed me that it was called Lord Roberts. Like Cary Grant cradling his adopted child in *Pennies from Heaven,* I took little Lord Roberts home to my wife and, with much ceremony, mulching, and patting, we put it to bed.

Twenty-seven years later, I am deep in the oblivion of a hard-earned Sunday afternoon nap when the front doorbell rings. No one else is home. Dressed only in a T-shirt and khaki shorts, I slip into my sandals and pad grumpily to the front door. I open it to find standing before me a tall overweight young man in a three-piece suit. As Yogi Berra would say, "It's dé jà vu all over again."

Half-asleep, I nod understandingly and say, "Let me guess—you're about to praise the Lord Roberts."

"No, sir," he smiles, handing me a pamphlet, "just the Lord."

RULE 10:

Never Complain That Hospital Food Is Hard to Swallow

I have a recurrent nightmare that I've been admitted to a hospital where I choke on my first bite of scrambled egg substitute. A nurse reports my failed gulp to my internist who promptly calls my HMO for advice. A 17-year-old clerk instructs my internist to order a swallowing evaluation on me. I wake up screaming and gagging.

There are few things more uncomfortable or frightening than difficulty swallowing. One of these things is a hospital swallowing evaluation. Among the common symptoms of old age (besides fatigue, shortness of breath, and achy joints) is difficulty swallowing—"dysphagia," as doctors call it. Like other symptoms, dysphagia ranges from mild to severe and has numerous causes, from a nervous tightening of the throat to a stroke-induced impairment of the swallowing muscles. Accordingly, treatment can be as simple as not talking while eating or as drastic as implanting a permanent feeding tube.

When patients with a stroke or Parkinson's disease choke a bit while eating, they may invite the rough embrace of the Heimlich maneuver with their next swallow or the agony of aspiration pneumonia. Or they may not. For some reason, hospital personnel tend to overreact when a patient swallows the wrong way for the first time. They choose to ignore Aristotle's observation that one swallow does not make a summer. If a hospital patient so much as hiccups while swallowing, he may precipitate a Grenada-like invasion of his privacy by an army of high-tech special forces.

Let me illustrate the horrors of this invasion, otherwise known in hospital lingo as a Swal Eval. My patient, whom I will call Mr. Milton Levy, is a 93-year-old gentleman who has just suffered his third stroke. He's a little weak on his left side but can still talk.

"How's it going, Milton?" I ask one morning before I examine him.

"Horrible, terrible."

Since he's been saying the same thing since his first stroke in 1971, I write "condition stable" in his chart notes.

He shakily picks up his cardboard cup of water, takes a sip, and begins coughing. A cleaning lady, recently arrived on these shores from Cambodia, looks up from her mop and pail across the room and announces, "Mr. Levy, he no can swallow water!"

Mr. Levy continues to cough, attracting the attention of the head nurse who happens to be passing by the room. "What's the problem here?" she asks.

"He no can swallow water!" says the cleaning lady.

"What she's trying to say," I point out to the head nurse, "is that Mr. Levy suffers a bit of dysphagia during the deglutition of water."

"What *you're* trying to say," instructs the head nurse, "is that this patient needs a Swal Eval!"

Oh no! I've done it again—let myself get trapped into ordering a swallowing evaluation. Once the head nurse suggests a Swal Eval, how could I be so hard-hearted as to let Mr. Levy choke to death on his next sip of lukewarm water?

Very reluctantly, I put him on NPO (nothing by mouth), start him on intravenous fluids, and order a swallowing evaluation. I have just unleashed on sweet, gentle Mr. Levy a speech therapist, an otolaryngologist, a neurologist, and a radiologist. One minute, he sits comfortably neglected and bored out of his wits and the next, he's got four subspecialists who can't wait to get their hands around his throat.

The swallowing evaluation involves finding out why Mr. Levy has trouble swallowing and seeing if there's something that can be done about it short of inserting a feeding tube. To my surprise, HMOs encourage Swal Evals, since they can theoretically prevent aspiration pneumonia, a very expensive disease. In the pre-Managed Care days, I would simply order thick liquids instead of water and often as not, the patient could swallow normally without a Swal Eval. Nowadays such a hit-and-miss approach is considered potentially costly and therefore risky.

The Eval begins with the speech therapist, usually a highly motivated, intense young woman, who strenuously enunciates her words. Next time I walk into the room and ask, "How's it going, Milton?" she frowns up at me from her bedside chair. "I'M SORRY,

DOCTOR," she informs me with a great deal of facial English, "BUT WE'RE IN THE MIDDLE OF A SWAL EVAL."

"WELL," I enunciate back, "EXCUUUSE ME!"

The speech therapist offers Mr. Levy a succession of increasingly viscous substances to swallow, beginning with water, moving to syrup, and ending with a cookie. Mr. Levy obliges by choking vigorously on the proffered sip of water, but not at all on the syrup or the cookie.

An otolaryngolist is called in. He shines an indirect laryngoscope down Mr. Levy's throat and asks him to say the letter "E." With that metal tube inside his mouth, Mr. Levy's "E" comes out "Oy." The patient then begins to cough around the instrument. "Hyperactive gag reflex," writes the otolaryngologist in his chart notes. The Swal Eval is proceeding nicely.

Enter the bearded and brawny neurologist. After introducing himself, he orders Mr. Levy to raise both his hands. "Please," offers the patient, attempting to comply, "my wallet's in the bedside table."

"We'll get to that later," smiles the neurologist whose reduced fee under Managed Care will top out at $200 for this five-minute visit. "I just want to see if you're weak on one side." In the end, the neurologist confirms that the patient has indeed had a stroke and possibly may be at risk for aspiration.

Then it's off to the radiology department for Mr. Levy, who will play a starring role in a three-minute genre motion picture known as a swallowing videofluoroscopy. The title of this brief but poignant film is called *Gagging Mr. Levy.* During the videofluoroscopy, several viscosities of barium are offered to Mr. Levy: the first is watery, the second soupy, and the third is a vanilla wafer coated with barium paste.

The radiologist, whom I've always accused of being a frustrated film director, enters the room brandishing a megaphone. He tells me he uses the megaphone because most of the patients sent in for a swallowing evaluation are elderly and hard of hearing.

"Then why the canvas-backed chair, the beret, and the black shiny boots?" I ask. "Add a monocle and you're Eric von Stroheim."

"Cool it, Oscar," he says, "we're in the middle of a Swal Eval and I don't want to go over budget." He then screws in a monocle.

"Aha!" I cry.

"Quiet on the set!" he orders, then shouts into Mr. Levy's better ear, "When I say 'Action,' *svallow* the *vasser!* Lights, Camera, Action!" On cue, Mr. Levy swallows the watery barium and promptly chokes.

What a trouper! He then is screen-tested while trying to swallow the soupy barium, and, for dessert, the coated cookie.

In the darkroom, the video tapes are examined by the radiologist as minutely as the Zapruder film by an assassination buff. After a couple of days, with Mr. Levy still on NPO and I.V. fluids, the swallowing evaluation team issues a joint diagnosis: Dysphagia for Thin Liquids.

The evaluation has cost $1,823 and the cleaning lady from Cambodia made the diagnosis for nothing! ("Mr. Levy, he no can swallow water!") The upshot of the Swal Eval is that Mr. Levy finds the only thing he can swallow comfortably is a vanilla wafer coated with barium paste. The uncoated cookie sticks in his throat.

By this time, the Swal Eval is totally out of my hands. The next day, under the guidance of his HMO, Mr. Levy is transferred to a nursing home with a gallon of lemon-flavored barium paste and a dozen cartons of vanilla wafers. The following week he is readmitted to the hospital for a Constipation Eval.

Why, you might ask, should I get all fired up over a measly Swal Eval when Managed Care is threatening to ingest, whole, the private practice of American medicine? Before Managed Care engulfs and devours our health care system, I modestly propose that what Managed Care needs is a Swal Eval.

RULE 11:

Nothing Confounds Death More Than a Loving Spouse

The most defining characteristic of Managed Care is its lack of compassion. You can't survive Managed Care alone. You need a partner, preferably a loving spouse, who can save your dignity when doctors fail to save your life.

In 1958, during my first year of medical school at Missouri University, our class was required to attend a series of lectures on syphilis. Our teacher was a member of a dying breed of academic physician known as a syphilologist. Professor Austin Ellis was an aging relic of the pre-penicillin Dark Ages of American medicine.

When he was a medical student syphilis was still destroying millions of men and women, and nothing could stop it. All medicine could do was describe it.

Syphilis attacked every organ in the body and quickly gained a reputation among diseases as "The Great Impersonator." Through its primary, secondary, and tertiary stages, it could resemble anything from a common cold to a brain tumor. Professors like Ellis were fond of saying, "If you know syphilis, you know medicine."

Ellis knew syphilis. He needed hundreds of thousands of words to describe its varied manifestations and only one word to describe its cure: penicillin. He never mentioned that one word. By 1945, when it came into widespread use, penicillin not only sounded the death knell for syphilis, but for the syphilologist as well. Despite penicillin, syphilis still lives a fugitive life, but you would be hard put to find a surviving syphilologist.

Alexander Fleming's fortuitous discovery of penicillin in a mold "contaminating" one of his bacterial culture plates remains the most dramatic and transforming event in the history of medicine. Like other bacteria, the spirochete of syphilis miraculously swells and bursts when touched by penicillin. Equally astonishing, the spirochete of syphilis, unlike other bacteria, has never developed resistance to penicillin.

By 1958, penicillin had been used extensively for 10 years and had virtually rendered Professor Ellis obsolete. Syphilis was rapidly being downgraded from a scourge of humanity to a medical curiosity. Still, Ellis's voluminous notes on the disease had themselves proved resistant to penicillin and we medical students were forced to learn them.

At the time, Dr. Ellis was a man in his early 60s. He was tall and portly and had a flushed face and bulbous nose. When he lectured, he kept his right profile turned toward us in order to hide a large scar below his left ear where his parotid gland and part of his upper jaw had been removed in a cancer operation about five years before we met him. His thick white hair was beautifully groomed as if to compensate for the disfiguring scar.

An aloof and harried man, he spoke with a high-pitched and slightly pompous voice reminiscent of W.C. Fields. He still seemed afflicted with the self-importance of the pre-penicillin syphilologist, who had been lord and master over three wards of dying patients. Now he was lucky to be asked to consult on two or three patients a year. Unlike those of most of our professors, his long white coat was spotless and neatly pressed, suggesting he had a fastidious and caring wife.

We were 44 young men plus 3 young women, seated restlessly in an overheated lecture hall in the dead of Missouri's winter of 1958, forced to listen to an obsolete professor discourse at length on a rapidly fading disease. From his opening remarks, we sensed that something was wrong with our professor.

He recited an anecdote involving the Italians of the sixteenth century who referred to syphilis as "the French disease," while the French in turn described it as "the Spanish disease." It was a good ice-breaker and we laughed appreciatively, only to be mystified a few moments later by his repetition of the same anecdote as if he had never told it to us. Our laughter the second time around was politely subdued and punctuated by an occasional snicker.

Ellis abruptly turned to his thick stack of note cards and read somewhat haltingly from them until the close of the hour. He allowed no time for questions from the class.

As the weeks inched by, his voice began trailing off as he read from his notes. From time to time, he would look up and stare vacantly through the frost-edged windows of the lecture hall at the snow-clad campus. After about 30 seconds, our scuffling shoes on the hardwood floor brought him back from his reverie with a start, and he would read us another horror story about the manifestations of tertiary syphilis.

One memorable Tuesday morning, he paraded before the class two patients "borrowed" from a nearby mental institution. Dr. Ellis's live demonstration of tertiary neurosyphilis was the annual pièce de résistance of his lecture series.

Seated on wooden chairs near the podium, the thin, pale men, both in their mid-50s, were dressed in freshly laundered overalls and work shirts. They were imperfectly shaven for the event—bits of bloody toilet tissue adhered to their faces. Their long dark hair was still wet from their morning shower and was slicked back from hasty combing by their nurses.

The patient on our left looked over the class with an idiotic grin, which, in retrospect, was not an inappropriate response to 47 first-year medical students staring at him in open-mouthed wonder. The other patient wore the saddest facial expression I had ever seen.

Professor Ellis briefly interrogated the first patient. Still grinning, the patient babbled nonsense when asked to recite his name, the day of the week, and where he was born. Professor Ellis reminded him (incorrectly) that the day was Wednesday. He then asked the second patient to walk the length of the room. Grotesquely, the patient with the Emmett Kelly face planted his shoes a yard apart and began waddling slowly toward the door. After a few steps, he turned to us and, in a cheerful voice that belied his mournful countenance, said, "Bet you folks ain't never seen no one walk like this before!" After being trotted out for 10 years, he had become a trouper in the medical sideshow of tertiary syphilis.

Clumsily assisting the patient back into his chair, Dr. Ellis turned to the class and observed, "The classic, broad-based gait of paresis." Even we benighted freshmen knew that Professor Ellis had confused the two patients: it was the first one who suffered the dementia of paresis and the second who rocked with the classic gait of tabes dorsalis. We learned later from our textbooks that the second patient's aggrieved expression was also characteristic of tabes dorsalis.

Dr. Ellis nodded toward the door and two beautiful young nuns blushingly entered the room to return the patients to their hospital. "Let's go, Harry," softly urged the first nurse to the grinning patient, who seemed reluctant to leave. "Easy does it, George," said the second nun to the wildly swaying patient on her arm. It occurred to me that if the two men had met similar visions of loveliness and virtue when they were about to sow their wild oats as young men, they would have been spared wasting the second half of their lives as museum exhibits.

When the men and their escorts left the room, Dr. Ellis pointed to one of our classmates whose hand was raised. "Professor Ellis," he asked, "would giving those patients penicillin at this time help at all?" The student had the effrontery to use the "P" word with the syphilologist. Dr. Ellis huffily responded, "No, much too late. They both received large doses and it didn't help them a bit. Next question."

Thirty hands shot up, startling the dazed professor. "If there are no further questions," he mumbled, "class dismissed."

Most of us had not been so much disturbed by the ghastly disabilities of the two patients as by the progressive befuddlement of Dr. Ellis. One of our classmates, Walter Gates, was a former pastor who had received, as he put it, a call to medicine from God at age 40. The rest of us had received a call to medicine from our mothers at age 13. Walter was our freshman father figure. After class that day, Walter announced, "Ellis needs help. I'm going to have a talk with the Dean."

The outcome of Walter's talk was that Dean Matthews quietly insinuated himself in the back of the lecture hall before Professor Ellis began his next lesson. Apparently, cardiovascular syphilis was Ellis's first love because, after a shaky start, he flawlessly delivered, without using his notes, a most informative lecture on syphilitic aneurysms of the aorta! We were stunned. When the chips were down, Ellis had rallied to give us his finest hour.

Dean Matthews was irritated at having been asked to spy on a fellow member of the faculty who obviously was far from being *non compos mentis*, as our father figure had described him. "He's not the old Ellis, I grant you," said Dean Matthews, "but he looks to me as if he's got quite a lot of mileage left in him."

The next day, Dr. Ellis relapsed into his confusional state. He not only slurred his sentences but seemed to drag his right leg slightly when he walked to the blackboard. His handwriting with a stick of chalk was unreadable. Inadvertently, he gave us future doctors our first lessons in opaque penmanship.

Day by day he seemed to worsen. We were forced to attend each class because the questions on his infamously difficult final exam were to be taken solely from his lecture notes and not from our textbooks. We were the captive audience of an impaired professor whose confusion threatened to flunk the lot of us. Poorly suppressed hoots of derision began greeting his incoherent statements.

Finally, Walter decided to call Mrs. Ellis and ask her if she had noticed any obvious decline in her husband's health. She said that, except for his seeming a bit more quiet lately and going to bed earlier than usual, she had not been aware of anything out of the ordinary. Walter ended his conversation with Mrs. Ellis by urging her to attend one of her husband's lectures. Walter said he spoke for the rest of us in believing that the professor had not only lost his ability to teach, but was in urgent need of medical care. Expressing disbelief, she agreed to attend his next lecture.

It was one of those marrow-freezing, mid-winter Missouri mornings. Ten minutes late, Professor Ellis shuffled red-cheeked and purple-nosed into the classroom and struggled out of his smartly tailored, black woolen coat. He slowly unwrapped a white silk scarf from his neck as if it were a bandage over his brutal scar. After tremulously hanging coat and scarf on a wall hook, he asked that the room lights be dimmed in order to project some slides he had brought with him. During the darkened interval, Walter Gates quickly escorted Mrs. Ellis, also dressed in a black coat, to a seat at the rear of the lecture hall.

"May I have the first slide, please?" asked Dr. Ellis.

On the screen appeared a colored picture of a patient extending the palms of his hands to illustrate the rash of secondary syphilis. Without looking at the slide, Professor Ellis squinted and read from a note card illuminated by a small lamp over his lectern: "The chancre of primary syphilis, uh, is usually found on or around the external genitalia but here we, uh, see a chancre of the tongue. Next slide, please."

For 15 minutes, Professor Ellis proceeded to read descriptions of the various stages of syphilis that bore no resemblance to the projected slides. Sometimes he read the same note card twice. He began stumbling over every other word. He frequently adjusted his dentures with his thumb and wiped the lenses of his glasses with a handkerchief.

When a portrait of the sad-faced patient we had recently met in our classroom appeared on the screen and Professor Ellis identified him as "a six-year-old boy with the classic Hutchinson teeth of congenital syphilis," his wife stood up in the back of the room and asked, "Will someone please turn on the lights?"

Professor Ellis blinked in perplexity and again wiped his glasses on seeing his wife approach him. With tears in her eyes, the slim, attractive, silver-haired lady walked up to the lectern and said, "Austin, it's time to go home."

Professor Ellis glanced at his watch and said, "Well, I'll be—so it is!"

Refusing Walter's efforts to assist her, she removed her husband's overcoat and scarf from the wall hook and helped bundle him up for the walk to their car. The professor offered no protest. Arm in arm, the two black-garbed figures made their stately way out of the classroom.

As soon as the Ellises had disappeared, Walter Gates stood up and addressed his guilt-stricken classmates. "Well, we've just witnessed the end of an era—and of a gentleman."

Dr. Ellis died a week later on the operating table while a neurosurgeon attempted to remove a large brain metastasis from his parotid cancer.

Professor Ellis had taught us almost nothing of the three stages of syphilis but almost everything about the seventh age of man:

"...second childishness, and mere oblivion, sans teeth, sans eyes, sans taste, sans everything."

Sans everything, that is, but his wife's love, which had cloaked his exit with dignity.

And now, 37 years later, I've admitted my ninth patient with AIDS to our local hospital. I've turned his care over to a specialist in Infectious Disease—a young Ellis—who will extract much data from him and, in the end, provide him only with comfort. Meanwhile, the patient's family and friends will administer the intensive care of love, hoping for that blessed day when another Fleming will routinely lift the lid of a culture dish impregnated with HIV and say, "Hello? What's this?"

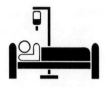

RULE 12:

Your Doctor May Be Able to Save Your Life, but Can He Remove Your Earwax?

W hen I retire from the practice of internal medicine—I've been at it for 33 years—my patients will remember me for just two things: I always returned their phone calls and I often removed their earwax. Of course, before I can retire, I might gratefully drop dead while filling out a patient's disability form, in which case I won't have returned all my phone calls that day. That leaves about 17 pounds of earwax as my monument.

In the matter of earwax, Managed Care and I see eye to eye. To contain costs, Managed Care would rather have me try to remove your earwax than send you off to an expensive ear, nose, and throat specialist. By agreeing with this policy, I don't want Managed Care to think that I'm extending an olive branch or even a Q-tip. I remove earwax to please my patients, not their HMOs.

Before you dismiss the removal of earwax as a trivial pursuit, let me remind you that we internists don't perform many procedures— for the most part, we serve as diagnosticians and non-surgical therapists—so we welcome an opportunity to play surgeon from time to time on an earful of wax.

How I envy the surgeons! Their patients are so dramatically cured and so grateful. In an ophthalmologist's office, they cry, "I can see!" In a urologist's office, they shout, "I can pee!" In an orthopedist's office, they yell, "I can walk!" In my office, if I'm lucky, they grunt, "Eh."

When I ask an elderly gentleman with an irritable colon how he's doing since I prescribed a tablespoon of psyllium husks in water each morning, he rewards me with a shrug of his shoulders and a less than heartfelt, "Eh." If I'm having a bad day and the patient is having a worse one, he will favor me with an "Oy."

How I envy the surgeons! I love what the British humorist Evelyn Waugh said when he learned that Randolph Churchill, Winston's brilliant but very difficult son, had a benign tumor removed from his lung: "Leave it to the surgeons to find the only thing that was benign in Randolph and remove it."

So perhaps you can see how thrilled I am when a patient comes into my office holding his right ear and loudly proclaiming, "Doc, I've got this terrific stuffiness in my ear that's killing me! I'm deaf as a doorknob!"

With trembling hands, I shine the light of my otoscope into his auditory canal and discover—Eureka!—a solid wall of earwax or "cerumen" as we doctors call it, if we expect to get paid for removing it.

I alert my overworked secretary, Jackie, to fill up a pitcher of warm water and bring me my giant warm-water syringe and my small metal ear probe. (For some reason, Jackie does not share my enthusiasm for the imminent procedure.)

Draped in a paper gown like a customer in a barber shop, the patient sits expectantly on the edge of the examining table. He flinches as I approach him with a 10 X 3-inch steel syringe. Ordering him to relax, I squirt a powerful jet of warm water into his right ear canal. Then I tug at the plug of cerumen with my metal probe and look inside. What I see causes me to rock back on my heels in alarm. I am reminded of the scene in *Raiders of the Lost Ark* when a boulder the size of the EPCOT dome comes hurtling down on the hero. That's what the loosened ball of wax looks like through the magnifying lens of my otoscope.

Soon, the patient is gleefully shouting, "I can hear! I can hear!" To this beleaguered internist's delicate ears, these words are music indeed.

The strangest thing about earwax is—what's it doing there? The best guess I've been able to glean from the medical literature is that cerumen serves to discourage the growth of bacteria and the nesting of insects in the auditory canal. I hesitate to tell this to my patients, fearing they'll ask me to replace the cerumen or will start wearing earplugs until their canals again form a solid waxy buildup.

By the way, insects are not the strangest things doctors have removed from their patients' ears. Out of respect for your sensibilities,

I hesitate to disclose the nature of certain foreign bodies dislodged from ear canals by startled physicians.

Suffice it to say that, at the age of five, I had several dozen tiny glass balls washed out of my aching right ear. Over a period of several weeks, I had plucked them from a beaded lampshade in the living room of our apartment and was curious to see how many would fit in my ear. Forty-two. My doctor, as I recall, was vastly amused at my experiment. His merriment was not shared by my parents who were asked to pay $6.00 for the office visit before taking me home.

In 1940, this was an outrageously high fee and was the beginning of the snowballing costs—or as I term it, the waxballing costs—that have produced the current health care crisis. That's right, I am personally responsible for the entire mess—the whole ball of wax, as it were—known today as Managed Care. I must say I am terribly sorry.

Although earwax removal kits are available at drugstores, I don't advise your trying to remove large amounts of cerumen at home. When I first started treating earwax in my office, I was afflicted with the clumsiness of the amateur. I learned eventually that the water used must be hot enough to melt the wax, but not too hot or it will stimulate the patient's organ of balance in his inner ear and bring on an attack of vertigo. I often converted my exam table into a roller coaster until I learned to lower the temperature of the water and let cooler heads prevail.

Before I enlisted the services of an ear, nose, and throat specialist to teach me, I would tend to abrade the inside of the ear canal with my metal loop and cause a bit of bleeding. I also learned that a tiny branch of the vagus nerve innervates each of our ear canals. As a result, my overzealous squirting and probing often caused a reflexive cough.

Thanks to my early on-the-job training, a patient would leave my office coughing, lurching to the left from vertigo, and wearing a blood-stained bandage on his ear (the "Van Gogh sign," as my unworshipful secretary dubbed it). Despite these doctor-induced side effects, my patient would often be whooping, "I can hear! I can hear!"

Other doctors would be able to spot my patients at once on the busy street outside my office. Mine would be the ones who were lurching and coughing, displaying the Van Gogh sign, and unaccountably shouting for joy. "There goes one of London's cerumen impactions," my colleagues would say, shaking their heads until their own balls of earwax rattled like castanets.

It's a good thing for my patients and for me that I finally mastered the art of wax removal with no side effects. Long before the era of proliferating malpractice suits, I became flawlessly adept at what sculptors call "the lost-wax process." Otherwise, I'd be afraid of picking up the phone one morning to hear a malpractice lawyer announce in hushed, earnest tones, "Doctor, I represent Mr. Indiana Jones, one of your patients. You, uh, recently attempted to remove a ball of wax from...."

"Ah, blow it out your ear," I'd prescribe.

RULE 13:

Medicine May Have Changed in 2000 Years, but Patients Haven't

As an internist, I frequently must decide if a patient is truly sick or merely a hypochondriac. Recently a friend of mine, Professor Lynn Kraynak, referred me a patient who had been stuck with the label of hypochondriac for more than 1,700 years. The patient, Aelius Aristides, a public speaker and man of letters, was born in 117 A.D. in Greece, 2,102 years before the advent of Managed Care. Here was a patient I could spend some time with, as opposed to the five-minute drive-by workups mandated by Managed Care.

According to Professor Kraynak, a classicist specializing in Ancient Greec, Aristides wrote a great number of excruciatingly boring speeches, plus one remarkable work, *Sacred Tales*, in which he chronicled his numerous ailments and the treatments he received under the direction of Asclepius, the god of medicine. Lacking a touch-tone telephone, Greek patients in those days summoned Dr. Asclepius through the medium of dreams.

Professor Kraynak, who admits to being rather fond of old Aelius, pointed out that over the centuries scholars have written off her friend as a whining hypochondriac. The good professor pointed out to me, "Amazingly, we scholars have never gotten a medical opinion." She wondered if a modern physician (me) would be willing to examine Aristides' medical history and assess whether this patient was merely a *kvetch* (an ancient Greek term borrowed from the Yiddish to denote a complainer) or if he was really sick. She sent me a translation of *Sacred Tales* and thus I had that most important aid to a diagnostician: a detailed medical history. I readily agreed to take on the case of Aelius Aristides.

Presentation of a Case:

A.A., a 72-year-old Caucasian male sophist, has suffered from complaints of recurrent choking sensations, coughing, and malaise for the past 46 years. He apparently felt well until January 144 when, at age 26, he developed a mild sore throat after taking a warm springs bath in midwinter. Still symptomatic, he set out in freezing temperatures from his estate north of Pergamum to Rome, a journey that, due to illness, took 100 days instead of the customary 30.

En route, he developed discomfort in his ears, chills, high fever, loss of appetite, and shortness of breath. He also suffered from pain in his gums and was observed cupping his hands as if to catch falling teeth.

Arriving in Rome in the spring of 144, he was not yet fully recovered when he began complaining of abdominal bloating and a sensation of respiratory blockage in his throat. His Roman doctors prescribed a 48-hour purgation achieved by his drinking elaterium, a concoction whose active ingredient was squirting cucumber. He continued to ingest elaterium until he developed bloody diarrhea.

After this pharmacological approach failed to relieve his symptoms, a surgical consultation was obtained. Without anesthesia, surgeons made a superficial incision of the skin beginning from the patient's chest down to his bladder. Cupping instruments were applied to the profusely bleeding incision at which time the patient reported that he again suffered a severe blockage of breathing.

Still ailing in autumn, A.A. decided to return to his home in Asia Minor. Sailing from Rome, he suffered severe seasickness in the continuously stormy weather. But his dominant symptom continued to be recurrent upper respiratory blockage. "With much effort and disbelief, scarcely would I draw a rasping and shallow breath, then a constant constriction in my throat followed and I had fits of shivering.... Other things, which are impossible to describe, troubled me...." He states his doctors "were at a loss....There was nothing which did not trouble me."

"From such great origins," he wrote, "...my disease formed and grew, ever progressing as time went on." He was to suffer the rest of his life (about 46 years) with symptoms arising from his succession of illnesses contracted between January and November 144. His hopes of a great public career were dashed by his debilitating and voice-impairing symptoms.

He spent much of the remainder of his life as a patient at a Greek temple of medicine, the Asclepieum of Pergamum (by all accounts the Mayo Clinic of its day). His personal physician was none other than Asclepius himself, the god of medicine. Since Dr. Asclepius appeared only in his patients' dreams and thus issued his prescriptions while his patients slept, bed rest was the dominant activity, or inactivity, of Greek temple medicine. (Under Managed Care, old Aelius would be discharged to home care in three days, and his physician, Dr. Asclepius, censured for carrying around a caduceus instead of a stethoscope when he made rounds.)

A patient admitted for treatment to a second-century Greek medical temple was required to perform sacrifices and purification rituals before the heaven-sent doctor would appear. (In the same manner, a modern hospital patient, about to have his gallbladder removed, must first sacrifice a portion of his blood and urine, then submit to a vigorous purification of the operative site before the ethereal, gowned surgeon floats into view.)

A.A., like his fellow patients, was instructed by priests to lie down and allow Asclepius, the god of medicine, to appear in his dreams. In the morning, the patient would recount his dreams to a priest, who would interpret them and dispense what the doctor (Asclepius) ordered, in the form of medications, diet, and exercise. (This ancient interpretation of dreams by medical priests was the forerunner of modern psychoanalysis, just as the temple's low-calorie diets and grueling workouts anticipated the fat farm.)

Dr. Asclepius had his first contact with the dreaming patient in December 144. He ordered A.A. to bathe in the river during a strong north wind that same month. (A review of records of temple medicine in the first and second centuries has failed to disclose even one instance of a malpractice suit brought against Asclepius.)

A regimen of sleeping alternating with bathing followed, with no discernible improvement in the patient's symptoms. In the winter of 145, A.A. writes, "Body remarkably weak; bedridden for a long time. Three baths in river: rainy and stormy during baths. Undressed and dove into river in which rocks churned and timber was being carried along by wind and current."

When the patient emerged from this primitive version of a Jacuzzi bath, he reported feeling a warmth passing through his whole body while his skin took on a reddish hue. (There being no ability at the time to record body temperatures, one infers that the patient was either feverish or suffused with the ruddy glow often imparted by agitated aquatherapy.)

Despite these ministrations, A.A.'s condition worsened. He reported: "Flow from head... turmoil in chest... breath caught in throat, causing inflammation... constant expectation of death." He stated that whenever food touched his palate, the air passage would close, causing a choking sensation and a fiery pain that felt as if it were penetrating his brain.

In the summer of 145, his doctor prescribed medication in the form of soap mixed with raisins. Having overcome his initial resistance to a pharmacological approach, Dr. Asclepius proceeded to prescribe thousands of medications throughout the remainder of the patient's life.

During the summer, at age 27, he was prescribed numerous phlebotomies, in one case the blood being let from a vein in his forehead. With the nagging persistence of his complaints, his doctor told him, in effect, to jump in the lake or, at least, bathe in the river. The phlebotomies and the bathing eventually seemed to produce temporary comfort and relaxation.

In March 146, his doctor prescribed mud to be smeared on his body, followed by a bath in the Sacred Well. The next day, Dr. Asclepius again commanded the patient to smear on mud, but also to run around the temple three times. The patient complied, but "the strength of the north wind was indescribable, and the icy cold had increased." Heavy clothing was insufficient and the wind passed through and struck his side "like a spear."

Then he bathed in the Sacred Well (presumably surrounded by well-wishers). Afterwards, he and his comrades "passed the day like one in spring," not surprising since the vernal equinox had occurred a few days before on March 21.

Later in the spring of 146, at age 28, he could neither take nourishment, nor retain what he did take. On the advice of his physician, he rode a horse at dawn at full speed, during which time he felt somewhat better, only to relapse when he dismounted.

A year later, the patient was in need of constant attendance. He developed a constant, strong cough and fever. Dr. Asclepius diagnosed consumption (*Sacred Tales*, Vol. III, page 10).

Then in the fall of 148, he developed a very painful swelling in the groin that grew to extraordinary size. After four months, when the swelling was at its height, Asclepius prescribed a salty poultice. When applied to the mass, the poultice caused most of the swelling to disappear quickly, leaving an inflamed opening in the skin. The drainage site rapidly healed after the patient obediently smeared on an egg.

His health remained poor during 149 and was not improved by the two shipwrecks he survived that year. Once again, his doctor took advantage of the icebound winter to recommend that his patient bathe in the river. A number of spectators gathered on the banks to witness the by now famously sick patient take his cure. Curiously, when he emerged, he felt a "lightness throughout my body and a continuous body heat and contentment." This improvement persisted through the rest of the day until bedtime.

He awoke to 16 more years of recurrent respiratory and abdominal symptoms, culminating in his contracting signs of "the plague" in the summer of 165 at age 47. (An epidemic of smallpox at that time was later documented.) Dr. Asclepius prescribed a bile purge and the patient slowly improved.

On February 11, 166, the patient spent a routine day of bathing in the morning and vomiting at night. On February 13, he merely vomited.

By 170, A.A. found that work on his speeches, poems, and the recording of his dreams afforded him some relief from his continued symptoms. He observed that creative work made him oblivious to pain.

In 171, at age 53, A.A. hinted that he might be feeling somewhat better by noting that he had not bathed in five years, except rarely in the sea, river, or well, as prescribed by his aging physician. He continued to receive uncountable purges, enemas, and phlebotomies. Between treatments, he continued to write, speak, and edit with difficulty, but was able to work each day at least until midnight. He went barefoot in winter, slept in the open air, and wore no undershirt under his tunic.

The circumstances of his death in 189 or later are unknown. In fact, given his endurance and the absence of a death certificate, it is not clear if the patient ever died.

Comment:

Thanks to the careful recording of his symptoms in the *Sacred Tales*, this patient, who suffered more than 1,700 years ago, gives the physician of 1996 some insight into his actual diagnoses.

Historically, the patient, Aelius Aristides, has been written off as a whining hypochondriac. The second edition of the *Random House Unabridged Dictionary* strictly defines hypochondriasis as "an excessive preoccupation with one's health." Implied in this definition is the suspicion that the symptoms a hypochondriac suffers are largely imaginary or at least exaggerated. (I will call this exaggeration of symptoms the "implied definition" of hypochondriasis.) By strict definition, Aristides was indeed excessively preoccupied with his health, and therefore, a hypochondriac. But by implied definition, in my opinion, he was not a hypochondriac, because his symptoms were not imaginary or exaggerated, but truly gruesome, and clearly warranted "excessive preoccupation."

The elusive art of medical diagnosis is based largely on the patient's own story and secondarily on the results of physical examinations and laboratory tests. As a diagnostician, I am, of course, deprived of the opportunity to examine Aelius Aristides and order appropriate tests on him (may he rest in peace). On the other hand, I have a treasure trove of clinical information written down by the patient himself.

His repeated reference to a blockage of his upper airway passages, his choking sensations, and the burning pain in his throat clearly point to an inflammatory disease of the oropharyngeal cavity. More ominous, he developed high fever and shortness of breath, indicative of a lung infection. He then made the mistake (still committed to this day) of seeking medical advice.

Faithful to the standard practice of the time, his Roman physicians recommended purgation with a powerful drug called elaterium, derived from the squirting cucumber. Aristides, who proved to be a most compliant patient, took elatarium for two days before achieving the desired result of bloody diarrhea. Undoubtedly this massive purgation caused serious dehydration and a profound loss of vital minerals, notably potassium. The resulting hypokalemia (low blood potassium) produced abdominal distention leading to the infliction on the patient of another common treatment of the day—bloodletting.

His cough, chills, fever, and choking sensations can best be explained by invoking the diagnosis of pulmonary tuberculosis with spread to the epiglottis, a thin valve-like structure near the base of the tongue that protectively covers the upper airway during swallowing and prevents the entrance of food and drink into the larynx.

It is known that tuberculosis was prevalent at the time in the regions where the patient lived and traveled. In someone with

Aristides' hardy constitution (which he clearly demonstrated by surviving his midwinter baths and other debilitating therapies), tuberculosis can remain an indolent disease until the host's resistance is compromised.

I submit that the rigors of his initial, mid-winter journey to Rome, compounded by bloodletting and intestinal purges, significantly lowered his resistance to tuberculosis. The tubercle bacilli moved through his lungs, up into his epiglottis and eventually down into the lymph nodes of his groin. Small wonder he dismissed his Roman doctors and requested consultation with the Greek Asclepius!

According to the *Sacred Tales*, the patient developed a constant strong cough in October 147 and "the god showed that it was consumption." If my diagnosis of tuberculosis is correct, then Aristides' enforced horseback riding at full speed the previous spring is quite possibly the first recorded instance of galloping consumption. Are there any questions?

The innumerable symptoms that Aristides recorded make clinical sense to today's physician, at least to this one. The preoccupation with his health that he evinced in the *Sacred Tales* speaks more strongly for his having suffered from serious physical diseases than from hypochondriasis.

Aristides' relationship to his physician, Asclepius, I believe, is relevant to an appraisal of the modern doctor-patient relationship. Aelius Aristides' physician ministered to him while he slept. Asclepius, by any criterion, was a dream doctor—a physician who makes house calls in the middle of the night.

Aristides was, in some respects, a model patient in that he ascribed godlike attributes to his doctor and slavishly complied with Asclepius' sometimes punishing prescriptions. None of the drugs that Aristides reported taking is known by modern pharmacologists to cure. At best, these medications caused relief of symptoms largely due to their placebo effect; at worst, they caused new symptoms.

With a doctor who was a god to him, Aristides fully benefited from the physiologic effects of bed rest and placebo therapy prescribed by a trusted and worshipped physician (*placebo,* from the Latin for "I am pleasing"). A patient's expectation that any substance taken is going to be beneficial sets in motion salubrious neurohormonal and immunologic effects, whether the substance taken is inert or, in the case of poor Aristides, assertive.

Of great interest to me is the relief of symptoms this long-suffering sophist experienced while doing creative work—a function presumably of the pain-deadening effects of endorphins released from his central nervous system while he was happily absorbed in his writing. Aristides' experience inspires me to encourage my patients to lose themselves and their symptoms in creative pursuits.

In my own practice (begun in 1966, more than 1,700 years after Asclepius hung out his shingle), I tend to discourage slavish adherence to my recommendations and prescriptions. I try to encourage my patients to challenge me rather than adore me. Despite my entreaties, some of my patients persist in ascribing godlike qualities to me and take my medications as ordered without questioning my wisdom. For the most part, these worshipful patients do well, but when they do not, they tend to be profoundly disillusioned with their physician. Soon they are ascribing godlike qualities to their lawyer.

It's easy for the modern doctor to be condescending toward Greek temple medicine as it was practiced in the time of Aristides. Until the discovery of streptomycin by Waksman in 1943, the treatment of tuberculosis remained essentially the same as that in Aristides' day, namely, strictly enforced regimens of bed rest, bathing, prolonged exposure to the elements, and surgery to drain abscesses.

I predict that 200 years from now, physicians will look back at docs like me and our ancient gadgets (CAT scans, sonograms, colonoscopes) and our primitive therapies (antibiotics, open heart surgery) and have a fine dry chuckle. The doctor of 2190 A.D. will preside over a genetically engineered population conceived in petri dishes and programmed to be disease-free and eternally youthful after age 24. The doctor's role will be to encourage high-fat diets, smoking, sedentary behavior, and the unbuckling of seat belts in order to make room for the next, more perfect batch.

But let us return for a moment to the second century. Before the advent of a specific cure for diseases like tuberculosis, some patients got better, most did not. Many of those patients who were able to achieve remission of their infections before the antibiotic age undoubtedly benefited from the placebo effects of their medications and from a nurturing bond with their physicians, a case in point being that of Aelius Aristides and the doctor of his dreams, Asclepius.

Diagnostic Impressions

1. Pulmonary tuberculosis.
2. Tuberculous epiglottitis.
3. Tuberculous abscess of the inguinal lymph nodes.
4. Peptic gastritis or ulceration; possible gastroesophageal reflux with secondary laryngitis and epiglottitis.
5. Iron deficiency anemia due to multiple bloodlettings.
6. Dehydration, potassium deficiency and malnutrition due to multiple intestinal purgations.
7. Smallpox, age 47.
8. No evidence of unwarranted preoccupation with symptoms (no evidence of hypochondriasis).

Would Aelius Aristides have survived Managed Care? Yes. For one thing, he kept lean and well-exercised. For another, his HMO would never have approved his referral to a surgeon for bloodletting.

RULE 14:

When House Guests Peek into Your Medicine Cabinet, Make Them Turn a Sickly Green with Envy

For your edification, I fling open the doors to my hidden treasure: the jewel-like designer pills inside my medicine cabinet. Regard their pharmaceutical elegance! An amethyst capsule of Prilosec, an opalescent tablet of vitamin E—as beautiful in their way as Fabregé eggs. Under Managed Care, you will never see their likes again. If I can resist swallowing them, my precious pills will turn collectible in five years and be worth a fortune.

First, you'll see the aspirin. Not just plain old, crumbly 300 mg. aspirin, but tiny, shiny, 81 mg. aspirin. One a day prevents a fatal heart attack or stroke and possibly colon cancer.

Next, behold the TWINLAB Daily One Cap, arguably the most salubrious combination of vitamins and minerals ever jammed into a capsule almost large enough to make you gag. Besides minimal daily requirements of everything you'll need to stay alive till your next dose, it's full of the anti-oxidants, vitamins C and E. Along with aspirin, a Daily One Cap is a double-barreled shotgun defending you against heart disease and maybe cancer. As a bonus, it includes folic acid, an essential B vitamin that every teenage girl must take daily to prevent a ghastly fetal abnormality called neural tube defect, should she get pregnant in the future.

If you eat enough vegetables, grains, and fruit each day to stock half a bin in your local produce market, you won't need supplemental vitamins and minerals, including folic acid. I must admit, the vegetarians whom I treat have the lowest cholesterols, the fewest cancers, the smuggest expressions, and the greatest amounts of intestinal gas of any patients in my practice. You can spot them a mile away—skinny orange people with bloated abdomens, rather like relatively hairless orangutans, complete with a banana in hand.

One of the vegetarians once told me, "I never eat anything with a face on it. I'm into grains, fruits, and nuts. Yeah, I make tons of gas, but my farts smell like newlymown hay. May I demonstrate?"

"I'll pass," I replied, "if you promise not to. Young man, do you realize that your tons of pleasantly scented farts are contributing to the greenhouse effect and if you vegans don't start eating things with faces on them, you're going to die of heat exhaustion and drag all of us smelly carnivores down with you? May I demonstrate?"

Next to my Daily One Caps (each of which contains 150 mg. of vitamin C), I keep a bottle of 1000 mg. vitamin C tablets as a vitamin supplement to my multi-vitamin pill. I take an extra thousand milligrams of C daily in homage to Linus Pauling, who won two more Nobel Prizes than I have, and who took ten more grams of C daily than I do. Dr. Pauling believed that large doses of C prevented or delayed cancer. His death from prostatic cancer at 93 tends to suggest that one way to fend off the Big C is with the capital C.

In hopes I'll make it to 94, I also take an extra 400 units of vitamin E in addition to the 100 units in the Daily One Cap (if TWINLAB put all the stuff I wanted in one pill, it would be the size of a tennis ball). All my friends in cardiology take megadoses of E along with their baby aspirin. Besides, the sight of a glistening, golden pearl of vitamin E in the palm of my hand makes treating hypochondria a joy.

Further inspection of my medicine cabinet reveals office samples of Zantac and Axid, both H2 blockers, marvelously effective in relieving GERD, a condition I suffer from along with tens of millions of my fellow Americans. GERD stands for gastroesophageal reflux disorder, or heartburn with an attitude, and has become a hot medical topic in recent years. GERD is a major cause of chronic hoarseness and wheezing in older people (like me), and of aspiration pneumonia in even older people like my mother, to whom I mail samples of Zantac in exchange for refrigerated pastrami FedEx'ed from the deli section of Schnuck's Market in St. Louis. (Small wonder I need Zantac myself!) GERD may even be a cause of esophageal cancer, from which my father died at age 54.

On the second shelf you'll notice a bottle of Prilosec, an even more potent drug than Axid or Zantac in reducing the ability of the stomach to make acid. Instead of Zantac or Axid, I pop a Prilosec on those rare occasions I allow myself a late-night pizza (Mondays, Wednesdays, and Fridays). I usually have my mini-pizzas delivered and, on retiring, take a Prilosec to prevent what is known as "the Domino effect."

Prilosec, by the way, is part of a duet used these days to treat Helicobacter Pylori, a bacterium that, astoundingly, is the major cause of peptic ulcers. Along with Biaxin, a powerful and well-tolerated antibiotic, Prilosec is given for two weeks and, in most cases, the ulcer vanishes for good! Dr. B.J. Marshall, an Australian family practitioner, discovered this bacterial cause of peptic ulcer and, like many a pioneer in medicine, was laughed at initially and, like a precious few, honored eventually.

On the third shelf is Naprosyn 500 mg., which, when taken twice daily with meals, is probably the best treatment for acute pain in my neck, back, or limbs, short of a deep oil massage by Venus of Willendorf (as opposed to the digitally challenged Venus de Milo). I will not bore you with a list of my aches and pains, but, having never missed a day in the office after decades of practice, I am limping proof of the efficacy of an occasional Naprosyn or other NSAIDs (non-steroidal anti-inflammatory drugs).

Beware! If you're prone to hyperacidity, as I am, be sure to take a stomach protecting pill (Zantac or Cytotech) with your NSAID or you might wind up unconscious or dead in the ER with your face as white as Philadelphia cream cheese and your stools black as licorice whips. NSAIDs are notorious for causing bleeding stomach ulcers, especially in the elderly. If you take over-the-counter NSAIDs like Advil and Aleve, be sure to take something like Zantac or Cytotech, at the same time, to protect your stomach. Pepcid AC, Tagamet HB, and Zantac 75, all of which reduce stomach acid production, are among the latest of the prescription drugs to go over-the-counter.

Regard my box of Metamucil packets (smooth texture, citrus flavor) on the bottom shelf. Just as Prilosec, Zantac, and Axid work miracles in the upper intestinal tract, Metamucil, in my opinion, is the penicillin of the colon. Not only does this powdered psyllium help relieve both chronic constipation and diarrhea, but it tends to lower one's "bad" cholesterol. As they sing off-key in nursing homes, "Who could ask for anything more?"

For my elevated LDL cholesterol, you will find a bottle of Pravachol next to my box of Metamucil. Pravachol, like other HMG-CoA reductase inhibitors such as Mevacor and Zocor, holds promise of prolonging life by dissolving fatty deposits in the arterial lining, especially if combined with a drastic, low-fat diet. (Fat chance I'd stay on that!) It appears that Pravachol, by itself, can reduce the incidence of premature heart attacks by 60 to 70 percent (*American Journal of Cardiology*, March 1, 1995).

If I were chronically depressed, severely obsessive, or frequently panic-stricken, you would be sure to find Prozac or one of its cousins, Zoloft or Paxil, on the top shelf. Especially for people who are anxious as well as sad, Prozac can be as transforming as love at first sight. What some doctors call chronic fatigue syndrome, I call depression, and three bright-red tablets daily of Wellbutrin, an anti-depressant unrelated to Prozac, are as effective in waking up these people as Prince Charming's kiss was on Snow White.

Dexedrine or Ritalin can also produce spectacular, uplifting effects when used on elderly people who are nonspecifically pooped and achy—who, that is, feel "old." (For this imminent eventuality, I'm reserving a space in my medicine cabinet for Ritalin.) To help someone cope with the death of a loved one, small doses of Dexedrine or Ritalin during the day, and Xanax or Valium at bedtime, are among the best gifts this doctor has ever bestowed on a patient. After a month, I slowly taper these drugs to zero.

On the bottom shelf is a bottle of Tums 500. I take two a day as a calcium supplement—men need calcium, too—and to settle my stomach when my mini-pizza proves too much for the Prilosec.

Remember, before swallowing any of my medications, consult your PCP and PDR, PDQ (Primary Care Physician and Physicians Desk Reference) as soon as possible.

I sometimes dream that a Managed Care spy slips into my bathroom at night and I wake up to a medicine cabinet filled with generics. The horror! The horror!

RULE 15:

The Happiest Patients under Managed Care Are Doctors

Under Managed Care, the specialist is a dying breed and the generalist, a resurrected one. Young doctors finishing their training to be specialists are finding to their utter disbelief that no jobs are waiting for them. The gatekeepers of Managed Care are keeping the specialists in relatively solitary confinement.

In the course of just about everyone's life, there arises a dire need for a specialist. What happens when you suffer your dire need and your generalist can't find you a specialist, or your HMO denies your request to see one? You raise hell.

With the help of your generalist, you must fax, phone and Fed-Ex your HMO's directors until they open their rusty gate for you. Once inside the Managed Care enclave of endangered species, you can briefly visit one of the specialists who crouch semistarved in cages, like the duck-billed platypus at the Berlin Zoo.

On their way to extinction, quite a few specialists survive from the bygone days of fee-for-service. So you'd better hurry up and get really sick before your town runs out of specialists (or your HMO runs specialists out of town).

Last year, I was unlucky enough to need the services of an exceedingly rare breed of cardiologist known as an electrophysiologist. As a patient myself under Managed Care, I was delighted at being able to see this exotic specimen with almost no hassle—sometimes Managed Care can surprise you with its generosity. But perhaps my being a doctor helped me get elite service as a patient. My example may be the only reason to send your son or daughter to medical school. Sometimes that oily substance known as professional courtesy is the only grease that works on the squeaky gate of Managed Care.

I hope Managed Care treats you as well as it did me in my time of dire need.

If they shoot you up with enough morphine, you tend to forget that the tips of four long wires are tickling the insides of your heart. In a narcotic haze, you look up at a TV monitor in the small, equipment-jammed room and watch a heart fire off 180 beats per minute. A milligram more of morphine and you're almost amused to realize that it's your heart that's doing a Gregory Hines tap dance up there on the screen.

You become aware of a rapid pounding against the inside of your breastbone. You begin to feel weak, dizzy, and short of breath. You're about to panic when the commotion in your chest suddenly disappears. On the monitor, you watch your heart rate plummet from a scary 180 to a normal 72. A loud cheer erupts from the throats of two doctors and three technicians in the adjoining room.

Your drug-tinged, first reaction is, "I've got a heart full of hot wires and they're in the lounge watching football!" A minute later, you look up to see Dr. Lee smiling down at you.

"You're cured," he quietly announces. Standing behind him, his four assistants happily nod their agreement. It turns out, the football they were watching was your heart.

What's going on here?

In a word, "ablation"—to be more precise, radio frequency catheter ablation in a cardiac lab in Oakland. As I experienced it, ablation was a selective frying by remote control of a quarter-inch plug of my heart muscle containing faulty nerve fibers. Before they were fried (or "ablated"), these nerves had triggered my lifelong attacks of frenzied heart beats.

More than a million Americans are victims of unprovoked seizures of rapid heart action known as "paroxysmal supraventricular tachycardia" or SVT. I was lucky to be one of about 60 thousand patients to date whose SVT has been cured by ablation. Previous therapies involved lifetime use of drugs whose side effects included such mood-enhancers as constipation and impotence. Still, these side effects were tolerable compared to the agonizing symptoms of SVT.

Each bout of SVT not only took my breath away, but made me feel as if I would die at any moment if it didn't stop. During an attack, I would feel a dreadful churning in my chest; I would sweat profusely and almost faint if I stood up. The worst sensation was my helplessness to stop this runaway heart; it was indifferent to pills, prayers, and postural change.

After a few minutes—or a few hours—it would dramatically and suddenly stop, as unpredictably as it had begun. Every now and then an attack refused to stop, occasioning a nocturnal visit to our local emergency room, where one of my sleepy colleagues would give me an intravenous shot of verapamil, a rhythm regulator, that stopped my SVT cold (at a minimal risk of stopping my heart cold).

Then a week later I might lie back on my pillow for a Saturday afternoon nap and—BOOM—my heart would go bananas, instantly turbo-charging its rate from 72 to 180 beats per minute. My first reaction was always, "Oh God, not again."

There's one thing I'll miss about my former "heart attacks"—the celestial burst of joy that invariably followed their abrupt cessation. "Thank God!" I'd silently exalt. For hours afterward, I would revel in the utter sweetness of being alive and well. I almost feel sorry for people who go through life without suffering an attack of SVT—they'll never know the profound inner peace of a suddenly calmed heart.

We who were born with these defectively wired hearts have waited all our lives for a repairman and finally one has arrived—the electrophysiologist. This is a cardiologist who has mastered the intricate circuitry of the nerves that control our heart rate and rhythm. Normal hearts have a rate at rest of 60 to 100 evenly spaced beats per minute. In hearts whose nerves are shot due to birth defects or disease, the electrophysiologist can diagnose a wide variety of horrors. In some electrically impaired hearts, the rate can drop at any time to zero beats per minute, as seen in what is commonly referred to as "sudden death." Other hearts may instantly slow from 70 to only 28 beats a minute due to heart block, with resulting loss of consciousness. Still others, like mine, may speed to over 200 beats a minute.

Thanks to electrophysiologists, many of these dangerous heart rhythms can now be completely cured. Some cures involve the implantation of highly intelligent pacemakers that can speed up a slow heart, slow down a speedy one, and even jump-start a stopped heart. Other cures, such as mine, involve the pinpoint grilling of faulty heart nerves with the heat-emitting tip of a catheter threaded into the heart through a vein in the groin. With data transmitted by wires from my heart to his monitor, Dr. Lee painstakingly mapped the aberrant circuitry of my right atrium until he zeroed in on the exact spot to apply the heat.

Zap. Pause. "You're cured."

Declining Dr. Lee's suggestion that I wait a day or two, I was back at work the next morning. My secretary remarked at how frequently I seemed to bump into walls. Jackie obviously was not familiar with the signs of a morphine hangover.

Electrophysiologists not only cure patients, but they do it while sitting down in an adjacent room! This feat of Oz-like wizardry cannot be topped by even the best or longest-armed surgeons in the land.

I've enjoyed ten symptom-free months since my ablation. But there's still a 5 percent chance that my SVT will recur and then it's back to the old circuit board, or rather, off to see the Wizard. But in medicine, 95 percent is about as close to a cure as you can get.

To my delight and surprise, my HMO picked up the $10,000 tab for this procedure without a whimper. They must have calculated that an ablation was more cost-effective than a lifetime supply of medications plus periodic emergency room visits to tame my wild heart. They may have honored my being an HMO doctor as well as a patient—or found it cheaper to repair me than replace me. In any event, I'm very grateful.

Not enough time has passed to be able to say that radio frequency ablation will still be the treatment of choice for SVT in the future. This calculated heartburn may prove to have long-term, adverse consequences. For many who suffer SVT, chronic drug therapy seems to work quite well with minimal side effects. For me, on the other hand, ablation has been a godsend—American high-tech medicine at its very best.

Thanks to Dr. Michael A. Lee, the Wizard of Oakland, I feel like the Tin Man, presented in an elaborate ceremony with a brand-new heart.

RULE 16:

It's the Estrogen, Stupid

I don't want to sound too enthusiastic about the beneficial effects of estrogen for menopausal women because someone will point out that I'm not a woman and therefore should confine my remarks to that repulsive hormone, testosterone. In that case, did you know that the only true aphrodisiac for a woman is a dose of testosterone? I might also add that, being a man, I qualify as an expert in hormone deficiency since, like a menopausal woman, I also suffer from a relative dearth of estrogen. Perhaps you have already diagnosed my estrogen deficiency from the testy nature of my remarks.

For better or worse, I've been prescribing estrogen replacement to my menopausal patients for the past 33 years. I must have written over a thousand prescriptions for Premarin, .625 mg., and so far have not received any major complaints from my patients or one note of thanks from Ayerst Laboratories. Premarin, along with Lanoxin for heart failure and Synthroid for thyroid deficiency, is among the few brand-name drugs for which I do not recommend a cheap generic substitute, Managed Care notwithstanding. Premarin is made from the urine of pregnant mares, and I place my bet on the stables of Ayerst to outpace any other manufacturer of estrogen. Managed Care please note: Other types of estrogen are more likely to cause blood clots than Premarin.

During a woman's healthiest years (from her teens to her fifties), her body is flooded with estrogen. A young woman owes a large part of her excellent health and her beauty to estrogen. It's the defining female chemical, the elixir of her youth, the source of her excellent skin, her strong bones and teeth, her full head of gleaming hair, her distinctively swelled hips and protruding bosom, her enviably low cholesterol, her kindly disposition, her fetus-friendly womb, and (in case we men are still indifferent to her estrogenic attributes) her moist vagina and high-pitched, musical voice.

Take away estrogen later in life and what often stands before you is a sapped woman, fragile of bone, loose of tooth, thin of hair, sagging of face, sweaty of brow, drooping of bosom, dry of vagina, raspy of voice, irritable of mood, and narrow of arteries. She's tried calcium supplements, power walks, moisturizers inside and out, niacin, the Pritikin diet, and Prozac, and wonders if she's missed something. When I say, "It's the estrogen, stupid," she runs off to a naturopath who prescribes a "natural progesterone" that succeeds only in restoring her premenstrual tension. Managed Care should realize that a Premarin a day keeps the following specialists at bay: cardiologists, orthopedists, psychiatrists, dermatologists, and cosmetic surgeons.

If you carefully study the literature on the pros and cons of estrogen replacement, you will inevitably conclude that you're doomed if you do, doomed if you don't—cancer if you do, heart attack if you don't. After 33 years of examining women on and off of estrogen, I say, "Take it as if your life depends on it," as it often does.

Estrogen, like all hormones, affects every tissue in the body, not just the "target" organ, namely, the uterine lining. Estrogen exerts profoundly beneficial effects on the skeleton, the brain, and the heart. It's a protein builder, and when estrogen goes, so goes the protein framework of bone (crack!), and the fullness of muscle in face, torso, and limbs (slack!). Enter the orthopedic and plastic surgeons. Estrogen raises HDL, the "good" cholesterol, and lowers LDL, the bad, greatly reducing the incidence of premature heart attacks. There is some evidence estrogen protects against Alzheimer's disease and colon cancer. For many women it significantly brightens the mood.

Estrogen saves women from osteoporosis. No matter what you read about calcium supplements, estrogen is the mother's milk of female bones. I tell my patients, "You can gobble calcium pills and drink milk till the cows come home, and you'll still get osteoporosis if your bones aren't bathed in estrogen." Same goes for the beneficial effect of exercise on bones: a small benefit compared with that of estrogen, and too much exercise can thin the bones of younger women! In the elderly, the fracture of an osteoporotic hip is often a fatal disease.

What seems blindingly clear to this male observer of female patients for more than three decades is that menopausal women suffer a severe hormonal deficiency that may eventually break their bones and their hearts. Most of us men, on the other hand, continue to make enough testosterone after 50 to protect our bones—and, alas, break our hearts. Unlike estrogen, testosterone has an adverse effect on cholesterol fractions. (Why can't a man be more like a woman?)

Almost without exception, the women who have taken estrogen under my care for the past 33 years look and feel terrific. They have the best bones and cholesterols in town.

A number of women have pointed out to me that menopause is an act of nature and therefore should not be tampered with. I reply that floods, tornadoes, and earthquakes are also acts of nature, and are not so easily preventable as heart attacks and hip fractures. I suppose the nature theorists would argue that a forest fire is merely one of Mother Nature's hot flashes and one should try not to disturb her while she's having one.

It saddens me that militant anti-estrogenists, by scaring legions of menopausal women into shunning hormones, will recruit a barely standing army of bent, middle-aged draft-seekers, clutching their hearts and limping to a marching song whose words beg, "Open the window and turn down the heat."

Of course, not all menopausal women are destined to spend their golden years fanning themselves in coronary care units and orthopedic wings. Any woman over 50 could do worse than having her doctor measure her bone density and her high-density lipoproteins (her "good" cholesterol). If her cholesterol and her bones retain their high density, she can safely refuse estrogen replacement. Get these tests done fast before Managed Care decrees they aren't "cost-effective" (as compared to a relatively cheap, early grave).

What's that? Uterine cancer? Yes, no doubt about it, estrogen replacement slightly increases the risk of an easily treatable form of uterine cancer, which can largely be prevented by adding progesterone.

By the way, I also suggest that women take estrogen and progesterone daily to avoid the curse of a monthly period for eternity. Of course, if your uterus was removed you won't need the progesterone, just the estrogen. If your ovaries were also taken, you might need a bit of testosterone added to the estrogen to jump-start your libido. Don't wait too long to decide to take estrogen; a great deal of your skeleton melts away in the first two years after your last period. Bulletin: A new non-hormonal drug, Fosamax, may fend off osteoporosis almost as well as estrogen.

Breast cancer from estrogen replacement? Possibly, if you listen to the majority of investigators. Hell, yes, if you listen to the vociferous minority, some of whose data are pretty scary. Are you more likely to die of breast cancer or heart disease? Estrogen therapy clearly helps prevent premature death from heart disease, which kills 240,000 American women each year, and to some extent increases the risk of breast cancer, which kills 46,000 women. Take estrogen or leave it? Your family history of one disease over the other may help you decide which course to take.

Despite causing as much as a 30 percent increased risk of getting breast cancer, long-term estrogen replacement, according to Dr. Bruce Ettinger, a researcher with the Kaiser Permanente Medical Care Program, can cut a woman's risk of heart attack by 50 percent and of hip fracture by 75 percent.

Nothing is written in stone. In quality and quantity, studies of female diseases lag disgracefully behind those of male diseases. For example, we've learned a lot more about prostate cancer than breast cancer. It's well known that estrogen therapy will retard the growth of prostate cancer; not so well known is that estrogen therapy at times can shrink breast cancer. How else to explain the ten-year disappearance of widespread breast cancer in a 75-year-old woman whose doctor, as a last resort, put her on massive doses of estrogen in 1956? A year later, her cancer had simply vanished from her lungs, her bones, and her liver! I saw it with my own eyes on her X-rays. That was before doctors knew better than to prescribe estrogen for breast cancer.

With much crossing of fingers, prayers, and incantations, I recommend that women start enjoying the benefits of hormonal replacement therapy until further notice. Get mammograms and a pelvic exam yearly. Check your breasts monthly and have your doctor check them every six months. With these screening precautions, your chances of dying from estrogen replacement are probably much smaller than dying from a premature heart attack, stroke, or from a blood clot in the lung after the fracture of an osteoporotic hip.

Take estrogen and you'll look better, feel better, and live longer. If I'm wrong, you can come back to haunt me—by appointment only—but I'll probably have died by then of too much testosterone.

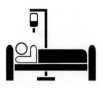

RULE 17:

Kill as Few Doctors as Possible

It may come as a surprise to learn that it's up to you the patient to keep your doctor fit for the rigors of practicing under Managed Care. Even though we doctors are trained from our first day of medical school to appear impervious to stress, please know that our skins are thinner than cling wrap. On my first day of medical school, I was introduced to a cadaver whose facial expression seemed to say, "Doc, don't just stand there, do something!" What I did was cut him dead, so to speak, but inside, my heart was bleeding.

Robert Weber created one of my favorite *New Yorker* cartoons. It shows a nurse greeting a patient in the waiting room, "The doctor will see you now, Mrs. Perkins. Please try not to upset him."

As a patient, you may not be aware of the immense power your every word and gesture has over your doctor. If you inadvertently upset your doctor, he may quite unconsciously change from your friendly physician to your grumpy gatekeeper before you can say, "Managed Care."

For example, never tell this physician, "Say, Doc, you look tired. Workin' too hard?" Whenever I'm told I look tired, I abruptly excuse myself for a moment, as if to finish resuscitating the heart of the patient next door, and urgently step into the office restroom to check my face in the mirror.

I pinch my pallid cheeks and hoist my downturned lips into my most beguiling smile. That fraudulently animated face staring back at me in the mirror doesn't fool me for a minute. I *do* look tired. I check my carotid pulse—whoops, an extrasystole! I dash cold water in my face, dry myself vigorously with a paper towel, and recheck my grinning visage. Countless tiny balls of white paper adhere to my five o'clock shadow; my face resembles a chia plant gone to seed.

Leaning forward against the wet sink, I massively stain the crotch of my gray flannel trousers. A slight pressure builds up behind my sternum and I loosen my collar. Through the narrowly opened restroom door, I reach out my hand. My ever-alert secretary, Jackie, pops her portable hair dryer into my palm like a surgical nurse handing off a retractor. With carefully aimed blasts of hot air, the dryer soon overheats the zipper on my fly, causing a mild, first-degree burn of my private sector. By the time I return to the patient's room, I am shouting, "Well, dammit, you don't look so hot yourself!"

As another patient sits on the end of the exam table, I crouch low to check her toes for Babinski reflexes. She looks down and comments, "Why, Doctor London, I've never noticed before, but you're getting a little bald."

"I am?" I ask, gingerly touching my pate.

"Yes, and I must say, it looks very distinguished."

As soon as I can extricate myself from the exam room, I ask to borrow Jackie's facial mirror and sequester myself again in the office restroom (the last refuge of a besieged doctor, until Managed Care installs surveillance cameras). Looking at the back of my head with the two-mirror technique, I confirm to my horror that the patient's diagnosis of incipient male pattern baldness is correct. I'm reminded, too late, of Satchel Paige's dictum, "Never look back. Something might be gaining on you."

Male doctors, and other self-appointed gods, are not impervious to the narcissistic wound of baldness. Caesar himself would have given up half of Gaul for a full head of hair—in his later years, Julius took to having his thinning locks combed forward and covering his scalp with an olive wreath, much as my Uncle Leon took to wearing a yarmulke late in life, to the bewilderment of his non-Orthodox family and friends. Well, I'm not about to perform a Caesarian on my thinning locks or resort to Uncle Leon's skullduggery!

Thanks to heroic scalp-reduction surgery, a half-gallon of minoxidil and strategically placed hair transplants, I have conquered my baldness. Actually, I overachieved. I now require the weekly services of a veterinarian to groom my locks. I have tendered my resignation to the Hair Club for Men and joined the Fur Club for Dogs. My surgically pointed head is topped by a small tuft of extremely thick hair which Doctor Horsely blow dries into a large puff that, although as fragile as a soufflé, covers my entire scalp. You don't believe me? Well, if you want to look down into a stare so withering it will curl your toes, try touching my hair while I'm checking your Babinskis. (As a relief from the horror story of Managed Care, I have just subjected you to a shaggy doc story. Forgive me.)

Another way to defeat your doctor without trying to involves coughing down the back of his neck, provided you are a male patient and your doctor is looking down as he checks you for hernia. As many of you men know, the hernia test requires you to stand up, turn your head to the left and cough while the doctor hooks a little finger into the right side of your groin to see if something bulges there. Now, the reason I ask you to turn your head to the left before coughing is that, if I didn't, you would dutifully cough down the back of my neck while I bend to my task.

The first cough usually goes well, dissipating off to the left somewhere. It's your second cough that gets me. When I hook my finger into your other side and ask you, "Cough again, please," often as not you will turn your head from the left toward the right and, while so doing, cough down the back of my neck, usually with more vigor than with the first cough, since by now you've gained confidence.

Why did you turn toward the right? Did I ask you? Are you trying to counter my threat to your dignity with one of your own to mine? Of course, what I should do to keep my neck dry is say something to the effect of, "Please keep your head turned to the left and cough again." Until I remember to say that, I'll remain wet behind the ears.

What I won't say is what one of my male heterosexual colleagues used to request during his exam for hernia, namely, "Give me a little cough, please." He likes to tell this story on himself: he once examined a handsome young fireman for hernia and to his horror and that of the patient, matter-of-factly came out with, "Give me a little kiss, please."

As we doctors are wont to say, "Hmmm."

God knows I try to make every encounter with my patients a therapeutic experience. But the adversarial stance some patients insist on taking toward their doctor threatens me with extinction at least three times a week. Lately, before walking into a hospital room to examine a patient, I insist that the patient's nurse and physical therapist accompany me. In this manner, I'm able to confront the patient and his family with reinforcements. What follows, in essence, is a tag-team wrestling match. A recent main event featured the London Angels versus the Klotkoff Avengers.

Mr. Herman Klotkoff, as I will call him, is a 78-year-old gentleman slowly recovering from a horrendous pneumonia. A powerfully built man who was formerly a scrap metal dealer, this old veteran of wrestling doctors into submission has until today been too weak to put up much of a fight. I've pretty much had my way with him, subjecting him to the gross indignities of intensive care. In the wrestling arena of his hospital room, he's either been flat on his back on the waterproof canvas of his bed or tied up in the ropes of his I.V. tubing. So far, he's been no match for the London Angels.

But now he has regained enough strength to take me on—he's recovering with a vengeance. He has signed up Leah, his long-suffering wife of the past 43 years, and Rosalie, his recently divorced daughter of 34, to climb into the ring with him. Together, this wounded lion of a man and his highly protective family comprise the Klotkoff Avengers.

With ingratiating smiles, the London Angels enter the ring and the nurse is immediately drop-kicked over the ropes by Mrs. Klotkoff's opening remark. "Why haven't you made up Herman's bed and refilled his water pitcher! Look at him—he's lying in urine and dying of thirst! Water, water everywhere and not a drop to drink!"

Slowly picking herself up from the ring apron, the nurse staggers off to refill the pitcher and gather up fresh linen. I'm left with the well-meaning, well-muscled physical therapist, Ms. Helga Hogan, to meet the challenge of the three Avengers. With his first words, Mr. Klotkoff gets a hammerlock around Helga's head and knocks her out on the ring post: "Don't come near me!" he shouts. "Let me alone! I'm too weak to walk! Let me die in peace! Out! Out!" Rubbing her forehead, a dazed Helga beats a zigzag retreat.

I suddenly find myself facing the Klotkoff Avengers alone! As the proud owner of the title, World's Best Doctor, I'm usually able to come out ahead in a one-on-one confrontation. But one against three? I'm a dead doc.

Behind me, the Daughter Klotkoff charges from a neutral corner and delivers a rabbit punch to my kidney with the announcement, "Dr. London, when you're finished talking to Mom and Dad, I've got some questions for you." I can feel my knees begin to buckle and my championship belt unbuckle.

Abruptly, Herman Klotkoff blindsides me with a flying cross-body block. "Doc, I wake up each morning cursing you for putting that totally unnecessary catheter in my bladder as soon as they wheeled me in. Ever since I pulled it out, I burn and hurt every time I pee. How could you do this to me! Don't get me wrong, I love you and am grateful for everything you've done, but why that catheter, you butcher?"

Before I can explain myself, Leah Klotkoff has me hoisted above her head in an aerial spin, before dashing me to the canvas with her accusation, "You forgot to order Herman a laxative and he suffered all night until I made the nurse give him an enema! How could you let him get blocked up that way!"

Herman Klotkoff promptly double-teams me with, "You doctors order antibiotics at the drop of a hat, but Milk of Magnesia? A patient could die first!"

Daughter Rosalie jumps in with a shock pinfall, "Question One—is Dad's HMO going to pay for his nursing care when he goes home?"

At this point, I give up. I am begging the referee, God, to step in and pull off the Klotkoffs, when Mrs. K. finishes me off with the observation, "Dr. London, you look a little tired. Are you maybe working too hard?"

Her comment is the verbal equivalent of the DDT, a back-bending, head-crushing finisher invented by wrestling immortal, Jake "The Snake" Roberts, who named it after the insecticide.

As I am dragged from the ring by the nurse and physical therapist who have returned too late to help me, I notice through swollen eyelids Sheldon Klotkoff, Attorney-at-Law, pacing the hallway just outside the patient's room. He is the young son of Fierce Demeanor, who had been waiting in reserve in the unlikely event his father, mother and sister had not been able to demolish the World's Best Doctor.

RULE 18:

Take Your Pills and Turn from Stud to Dud

As my old urology professor at Iowa used to say, "Any medication that gets into your bloodstream can fuck up your sex life." Blood pressure pills are the worst offenders. Often the patients don't know what hit them. Mr. Harvey B. has taken propanalol, a beta blocker, for a month and his doctor is thrilled to announce, "Harvey, your pressure's dropped 20 points!"

"So what?"

"That means you'll never wake up with a stroke!"

"Yeah, Doc—or a boner."

"What do you mean?"

"For the past month, my little richard has pointed south and stayed there. This morning, I caught my wife looking up 'gigolo' in the Yellow Pages. Fortunately, she was looking under J. What's going on here?"

"Well, it's possible the propanalol is causing a little erectile dysfunction."

"I'd rather have a little stroke."

"You mean to tell me you'd rather wake up with a limp arm and leg?"

"Yeah, I'd gladly give an arm and a leg to get my balls out of the freezer."

The doctor is dumbfounded that Harvey isn't bowing in gratitude and rather shocked by the bluntness of his language. After all, hypertension is the royal road to a stroke, the second leading cause of death. And the propanalol brought Harvey's blood pressure down from 200 over 95 to 130 over 70—normal, for God's sake!—and is the patient grateful? No, he's whining about a little erectile dysfunction, the ingrate. Compared to a stroke, this certainly is an acceptable side effect, isn't it?

Harvey says he'd rather die. "Doc, what does rigor mortis do for erectile dysfunction?"

"I don't know, but it wouldn't hurt."

The trouble with high blood pressure, also known as "the Silent Killer," is that the only symptoms it causes are the side effects of the drugs used to lower it.

"So, okay," the doctor concedes, "let's take you off the propanalol and put you on a mild diuretic for your hypertension."

In two weeks, Henry's blood pressure is still under control, but the patient is shaking his head and mumbling.

"Your little what?" asks the doctor. "Not that again!"

The doctor obviously didn't know that the "mild" diuretics commonly used for high blood pressure can also wipe out a patient's libido and I'm not just talking about male libido.

Both propanalol and HCTZ (the diuretic) are very inexpensive drugs, besides being very effective in treating hypertension. For these reasons, Managed Care loves them, impotence notwithstanding.

About the only blood pressure pills that seem to leave the sexual organs to their own devices are the ACE inhibitors (Vasotec, Zestril, Accupril, and others). These highly effective drugs cost a great deal more than propanalol and HCTZ. Mention Zestril to the chief accountant of your HMO and his blood pressure skyrockets.

Tranquilizers are another source of sexual angst for both men and women. Benzodiazepines like Valium and Xanax for daytime anxiety and Dalmane and Restoril for sleep have the power to reduce libido and, if you go for it anyway, delay ejaculation.

Besides chilling one's ardor, the benzodiazepines can also cause chemical dependency, withdrawal anxiety, danger of falling in the elderly, and forgetfulness. The side effects of Valium can create so much stress that it's a good thing the patient is taking a tranquilizer. Or am I missing something here?

Alcohol, unlike Valium, increases sexual desire, but, alas, blunts performance, creating a situation, especially after the age of 50, of high expectations in the barroom that peter out in the bedroom. A woman sleeping with a drunken man risks serious physical abuse if she chides him for his "hangover."

Anti-depressants cause the same problem. In my practice, the number of patients who suffer sexual dysfunction from the Prozac family (Prozac, Zoloft, Paxil, and their first cousin, Effexor) is scandalously high. In younger patients, delayed orgasm seems to be the problem (which could also be the solution to premature ejaculation). Older patients on Prozac have been known to tack notices on telephone poles describing their missing libido ("answers to the name Big Boy") and offering substantial rewards for its return. Some people taking Prozac, or one of its shorter-acting relatives such as Paxil, have learned that withholding that day's dose until after sex improves performance.

The original anti-depressants, the tricyclics, also knock one's libido out of the ball park. But, unlike the Prozac family, Elavil and others often cause dryness of the mouth, constipation, heart rhythm disturbances, and dizziness on standing up, which serve to take one's mind off one's sexual dysfunction. Impotence with Prozac is a lot more fun than with Elavil.

Headache remedies and other painkillers that contain hydrocodone or codeine can also banish lust. The age-old excuse for declining sexual overtures should be changed from, "Sorry, darling, I've got a headache," to "Sorry, darling, I just took a headache pill."

Pills that inhibit stomach-acid production like Zantac, Axid, cimetidine, and Prilosec can also cause dyspepsia of the sex drive. Absorbable drugs that lower your LDL cholesterol and your triglycerides, like Mevacor, Pravachol, Zocor, and Lopid, can likewise diminish your machismo and machisma. Between propanalol for your blood pressure and Pravachol for your cholesterol, you might remain alive above the waist, but find yourself dead below. To be fully alive, you might want to substitute Zestril for propanalol, and niacin for Pravachol.

Hardening of the arteries causes softening of the penis. Prostaglandin E-1, a natural body chemical, greatly enhances blood flow to the penis and is a wonder drug for impotence. One problem: the patient has to inject it through a fine needle into the shaft of his penis. For reassurance, a middle-aged man with impotence need only consult his teenage kids to learn that body piercing is "no big deal."

Since an erection occurs when much blood flows into the penis through tiny arteries, anything that constricts these arteries can cause impotence. Nicotine and caffeine might heighten the mood for sex, but through vasoconstriction, put a serious crimp in your evening's plans. Ergo, the ancient ritual of lighting up a cigarette after sex was probably learned the hard way.

RULE 19:

Suffer Gas Silently

When you sign up for an HMO that excludes your family doctor, you will soon find yourself seated in the waiting room of Dr. David Generic, who will treat you as if he never met you, because he hasn't. Didn't you realize when you switched to an HMO that you'd be giving up the man who delivered your children, saved your husband's life, and unnecessarily but deftly removed your son's appendix? It takes a number of years to bond with your doctor, attune your personality to his, and not be treated as a street person by his secretary when you ask for the restroom key. Would you break that sacred bond for lower premiums?

Your own dog, Roscoe, would never put up with a similar situation if veterinary medicine should ever switch from flea-for-service to Managed Cur. Over the years, Roscoe has grown attached—mostly around the ankle—to his vet, Old Doc Mange. It would be animal abuse to force Roscoe to switch to some cat-loving, thick-ankled vet. To express his displeasure, there's no telling what Roscoe might do on the carpet of the new vet's office before you could ask for the key to the litter room.

Your doc may be a quack, but he's your quack. Before you turn your back on your own quack, consider that after a few years of practice, doctors begin to attract their own distinctive type of patient. As a diagnostician, I can look out my office window in Berkeley and instantly match the pedestrians down below with their doctors.

For instance, Dr. Sidney Goldfarb's practice consists largely of professional whiplash injury cases. His patients limp slowly down the street wearing old, yellowing, foam rubber collars and schlepping cracked, peeling attaché cases bulging with insurance forms. The agony of having to care for this type of patient has caused Dr. Goldfarb himself to become rather bent over. "That must be one of

Sid Goldfarb's patients," a new doc on the block observes confidently. "No," I point out, "that's Sid Goldfarb."

I can see by the blinding light reflected from a number of prominent foreheads below me that Dr. Marcus Gottlieb's waiting room will soon be filled with Nobel laureates studiously ignoring one another. By contrast, Dr. Sheldon Bloom has cornered the Berkeley market in aging hippies—gray-bearded men, whose long hair is not holding at the center, whose open-toed sandals reveal nascent bunions, and who come to Dr. Bloom for minuscule doses of mycostatin for whatever ails them.

Dr. Bradley Atherton, on the other hand, specializes in diseases of the affluent. Striding aerobically, his patients are silver-haired Nordic giants afflicted with such *maladies d'élite* as Lacrosse elbow, wine cellar rhinitis, and Mercedes sunroof keratoses of the forehead (or MSRKF, as Dr. Atherton calls them in a paper he recently presented to his country club).

How can you tell my patients? Well, my patients are all lovely, of course, but tend to be overweight and suffer collectively from gas. They lightly bounce down the street, seeming to levitate a considerable distance off the sidewalk from time to time. On days when the barometric pressure is quite low, the sight of my patients marching toward my office resembles a Macy's Thanksgiving Day parade.

Some time ago, I discovered that a number of my gassy patients were addicted to carbonated water or, as it's called on the East Coast, seltzer. I promptly formed a seltzer support group. Over several weeks, I coaxed them from straight seltzer to Scotch and soda, then to Scotch on the rocks, and finally to straight Scotch. Then I turned them over to AA. That's one of the few ways I've been able to cure gas.

Whenever I'm asked how I like the practice of medicine in this age of Managed Care, I reply, "It's a gas."

Just before 5 P.M. in my office, I still have eight patients to see and 14 phone calls to make, and the phone rings and then rings again. My receptionist informs me that on line one is Mrs. Yetta Kamen, calling for the fourth time about her gas pains, and on line three is Dr. Harvey Mandell, an internist from Cleveland, whose aunt I have had hospitalized for the past week with fever and gas of unknown origin.

Mrs. Kamen is a frequent caller. She phones me at least three times a week and spends an average of 17 minutes per phone call. She and others like her have prompted me to initiate a frequent caller program in my office. After a patient has logged 500 phone calls, I send him or her a free airline ticket to Nome, Alaska. One way.

(In the past few years I've been besieged by patients begging me for notes to excuse them from flying on a certain date. For example: "Mrs. Yetta Kamen is too ill to fly as scheduled on March 4, 1996 due to gas pains that begin at 6000 feet." During the past two months alone, I must have written three dozen such excuses. When I learned that TWA had filed for bankruptcy protection, I felt personally responsible.)

Mrs. Kamen is still waiting on line one. Now, on line three is Dr. Harvey Mandell of Cleveland—one of my favorite phone calls— another internist calling from out of town about his relative and my patient. His calls are thinly disguised lectures on fevers of unknown origin associated with gas. Yesterday we discussed spontaneous pneumothorax; today he has scheduled a tutorial on "Febrile Diseases of the Descending Colon."

I don't know what to do with these two phone calls. Through clenched teeth, I tell my secretary, Jackie, to keep them on hold for 30 more seconds and then pull the phone wires out of the wall. This remark so unnerves her that she accidentally hooks Mrs. Kamen on line one with Dr. Mandell on line three in a conference call. Through the speaker on my desk phone I hear the following conversation:

MRS. KAMEN: Doctor?

DR. MANDELL: Yes?

MRS. K: It's the gas pains again. Now they're right under my heart. Please, Dr. London, help me!

DR. M: But I'm not Dr. London. I'm Dr. Mandell. I'm also waiting to talk with Dr. London.

MRS. K: You are? (voice drops to a hoarse, conspiratorial whisper) Listen, Dr. Mandell, as long as we're waiting together, can I speak frankly? Half the time Dr. London doesn't know what he's talking about. Maybe you can help me. In your opinion, what's good for gas?

DR. M: Have you tried the new Metamucil?

MRS. K: You mean the one without the grits?

DR. M: Yes.

MRS. K: I miss the grits. Anyway, Metamucil doesn't do a thing for me.

DR. M: How much do you use?

MRS. K: A teaspoon.

DR. M: Not enough. Try a tablespoon. Works like a charm every time.

MRS. K: You mean it? Thank you, Dr. Mandell! Please—send me a bill.

DR. M: I wouldn't think of it. Happy to help. By the way, what kind of medical insurance do you carry?

MRS. K: Forget it, Dr. Mandell. I'm in an HMO and you're not on my list of providers.

Mrs. Kamen hangs up. Jackie gets on the line and says, "Thanks for waiting, Dr. Mandell. Dr. London can speak with you now."

"Ah, forget it," says Dr. Mandell. "If what I just heard over your phone is what that poor bastard goes through every day, I won't bother him. Tell him to keep up the good work on my aunt."

There are moments before 5 P.M. when I could just pop—when a chic, but underweight lady comes to the window and complains about the mirror in my waiting room. "I've been out here for two hours, watching myself age visibly! Where's Dr. London?"

"He'll be with you shortly," says Jackie. "He's in the restroom taking a simethicone tablet."

Physician, burp thyself.

RULE 20:

Managed Care Would Have You Nibble Radishes at the Movies

The recent disclosure that a large box of buttered popcorn contains almost 2000 calories sent shock waves through the hearts of moviegoers. I suspect Managed Care, in its zeal to prevent admissions to the coronary care unit, is behind this popcorn exposé. I suppose the next thing they'll tell us is that a large box of Milk Duds is almost 500 calories. We cinema buffs don't want to hear this.

For decades, these calories were imbibed in darkness, exonerating the eater from blame. In the good old days before Managed Care, you were permitted to weigh yourself in a darkened bathroom when you returned home that night. This time-honored maneuver permitted you to tell yourself: "I can't see that I've gained any weight from all that junk I ate at the movies!"

I've been eating buttered popcorn at the movies for 50 years and if it's so bad, how come I'm still alive and almost all the movie stars are dead? Because while I was eating popcorn they were all smoking and drinking and God knows what else.

Just as they decree that you take generic drugs, Managed Care has sanctioned only air-popped, unbuttered popcorn. This tasteless fluff is no substitute for the real thing, though it is a substitute for Styrofoam pellets. What do they think my stomach is, a packing crate?

The only reason I go to the movies is to eat junk food in the dark. As a doctor, I can ill afford to indulge my addiction to Milk Duds, Jujyfruits, and buttered popcorn in broad daylight. If I'm seen in the doctors' lounge at Mt. Zion poking a Milk Dud in my mouth, I will be summoned before the peer review committee and stripped of my beeper. Besides, have you ever seen a Milk Dud in broad daylight? Let me assure you, it is not a pretty sight.

Until recently, the only other venue where it was politically correct to eat junk food besides a movie theater was a baseball park. Now word comes out of San Diego that in the grandstand of the Padres' stadium they have installed a sushi bar. I am not making this up. Before long, vendors will be marching up the aisles clacking chopsticks and hoarsely shouting, "Tamago! Ebi! Saba! Unagi!" A fan will shout back, "One Ebi! Two Unagis! Heavy on the soy sauce and hold the wasabi!" Managed Care strikes again.

Closer to home, a health-food bar has opened for business at San Francisco's Candlestick Park. I am not making this up, either. How can I enjoy my Polish dog and my Carnation frozen shake when one of my patients sidles up to me, nibbling a tofu burger, and demands, "Say it ain't so, Doc."

No, I must get my junk-food fix under cover of darkness at the movies. Incidentally, it's no fun eating movie food in the dark at home. This requires shopping for Milk Duds at the corner grocery, schlepping to Captain Video, popping my own corn, melting my own butter, fiddling with the color control on the VCR, settling back, slipping two Milk Duds into my mouth and hearing my wife shout, "WHAT ARE YOU TRYING TO DO? KILL YOURSELF?"

I attempt to answer, but the store-bought candy is so stale that my mouth is glued shut. I vastly prefer self-destructing with my fellow man at the movies, where my wife doesn't raise her voice and can indulge her own relatively mild addiction to Raisinets and M & M's.

Which brings us to the United Complex Odeon Galaxy Ten theater, where after waiting in a line that rivaled the Great Wall of China in length and immobility, we recently bought two tickets to *Forrest Gump*. By the time we got inside, it was moments before show time. When I saw that the Great Wall of China had reassembled itself in front of the refreshment stand, my heart sank.

Shrugging off her M & M withdrawal, my wife suggested we go into theater six at once and begin our fight to the death for two adjacent seats. But the thought of sitting without refreshments through a major motion picture now showing at a theater near me was intolerable.

"You go ahead," I said gallantly. "I'll get your M & M's and you find me a seat." Shooting me a glance that melted a shelf of Junior Mints 50 yards behind me, my wife abruptly left me for another man: a short, mustached usher who tried to open a path for her to theater six through a living wall of Siamese yuppies joined at the waist.

As the refreshment line inched forward, I explored my options:

Box of buttered popcorn—small, medium or large? Medium, of course. Actually, small is more than enough popcorn, but at $2.50 a box, why not spend 20¢ more and get the medium? After all, moderation in all things. A medium buttered popcorn is my choice and never the large! Once, I made the mistake of ordering a large box of popcorn, which required a large Diet Coke to wash it down. The next day I found it impossible to immerse myself in a tub of water. I floated high and largely dry on the surface, narrowing my rubber ducky's habitat to the slender estuary between my calves—a wholly unsatisfactory bathing experience for both O. London and R. Ducky.

Milk Duds or M & M's? Milk Duds, hands down. M & M's are so flawlessly made and immaculate to the touch that they come perilously close to transcending the junk food genre. When my wife proffers me one of her M & M's during a movie, I often as not swallow it whole with a sip of Diet Coke, mistaking it for a Zantac tablet. On the other hand, a lumpy, amorphous Milk Dud is quintessential movie food. A Milk Dud does not pretend to be a piece of Godiva chocolate, except in price.

A true movie junk foodie eschews the handsome bars of imported Swiss chocolates stacked like gold bouillon on the bottom shelf of the candy counter. Tobler's bars of pure milk chocolate with soft caramel centers are simply yuppie Milk Duds and no self-respecting cineplex should carry them. I have walked out of artsy movie houses that offer homemade chocolate truffles, for God's sake. As I see it, chocolate truffles are film festival food, not movie food.

A chili dog or nachos in cheese sauce? Both. Why waste precious minutes agonizing over choosing between these two lethal items, when you can have both for the price—severe heartburn—of one?

Warning: Chili dogs and nachos in cheese sauce are X-rated movie food. Raincoats are recommended. It was in a failing Jerry Lewis Cinema in El Cerrito 20 years ago that I first encountered nachos in cheese sauce being served to enchanted moviegoers. The theater closed down shortly after an audience of three people at a midnight showing of *Jaws* stood up to leave and couldn't. Our shoes were bonded to the floor.

But here I am 20 years later in front of a refreshment counter at a cinema complex and a teenage girl with chartreuse hair is taking my elaborate order, which breaks down as follows:

APPETIZER

A medium box of popcorn, topped with a shower of
melted butter, salted (4 packets) to taste

ENTREES

One chili dog, with onions, pickle, and mustard

One platter nachos in cheese sauce

DESSERT

Assorted Milk Duds, Jujyfruits, M & M's, Raisinets

BEVERAGE

One liter of Hawaiian Punch (Procter & Gamble, '95)

By the time the counterperson fills my order, her hair has
turned white, her braces have been replaced by dentures, and she
moves from the popcorn machine to the soda fountain with the aid of
a walker. Several people waiting in line behind me have died of natural causes. Meanwhile, the 7:00 P.M. showing of *Gump* is halfway
through the opening list of production credits. While waiting for her
to fill my Hawaiian Punch to the brim, I pry open the boxes of candy
and stealthily sample the contents.

With my food and beverage precariously balanced on two flim-
sy cardboard trays, I wheel about and make a tipsy beeline for the
napkin, straws, and salt counter. Just before reaching this halfway station between food and film, I trip over a vacuum cleaner being
manned by one of the ushers. Before I can ask myself what a goddamn vacuum cleaner is doing in a movie theater, I am airborne.

Were I a film director for this scene, I would use slow motion to
catch my sensual lips gradually widening in terror, the kernels of popcorn filling the air like flak over Düsseldorf, the progressive lengthen-
ing of the blood-red arc of Hawaiian Punch, the leisurely, missile-like
ascent of the chili dog, the steadily increasing atmospheric pollution of
Nachos, Milk Duds, Jujyfruits and Raisinets, the gentle descent of my
body like an ancient starship beginning an elaborate docking maneuver. The soundtrack would emit a deafening staccato wail as my sharp
utterance of a four-letter epithet slowly broke into its component
decibels.

But, lacking a camera and crew, I simply drop to the floor and
slowly get to my feet with at least 6000 calories clinging to my per-

son. At this juncture, my wife shoots out of theater six ready to chide me gently for dallyin. After perusing me clinically from head to toe, she plucks a flattened Raisinet from my forehead, pops it into her mouth and turns on her heel.

I profusely apologize to my wife and quickly order an emergency ration of popcorn, Hawaiian Punch, Milk Duds, and Jujyfruits before following her into the darkened theater. We watch what remains of *Gump* from two seats at either end of the first row. Two hours later we emerge from theater six with our necks stiff and twisted to one side and our heads fixed upward. Fortunately for me, we have to wear cervical collars for the next three weeks before we can make eye contact and I am saved her withering gaze.

I certainly agree with Mr. Gump that "life is like a box of chocolates. You never know what you're gonna git." Unless, of course, you order Milk Duds.

RULE 21:

Death Begins at 40

O ne reason Managed Care is so profitable is that it skims off the cream of the healthy, employed population who don't require much in the way of expensive care. Small wonder Managed Care is so gung ho about preventive medicine—by the time your well-conditioned but aged body begins to malfunction in parts not covered by your warranty, the CEOs of Managed Care will have long since retired to Palm Springs, Coral Gables, and Boca Raton.

Until we turn 40, we're all more or less gorgeous and seemingly immortal. During your 40th birthday party, may I suggest that you excuse yourself before you blow out the candles and step into the bathroom? Hop naked onto the scale and look in the mirror. If you have to take off your clothes to hop naked, you have not planned your party well. Be brave and behold. At 40, if you see at least 20 pounds more of you than you saw at 30, don't eat the cake. If there's a glass of gin in one hand and a cigarette in the other, put out the cigarette in the gin. The party's over. Managed Care begins.

Up till 40, you've been able, for the most part, to get away with anything. You are truly middle aged because you're halfway to 80, when, finally, what you do to your body isn't quite as damaging as what your body does to you—namely, reproduce your cells in a haphazard manner.

By 40, especially if you grew up in the Midwest as I did, you've eaten the equivalent of a fair-sized farm: in my case, 117 head of cattle, 812 hogs, 391 sheep, 13,212 fryers, 78 ducks, and 197 gobblers. (All those birds and animals died for me. And to whom do I send my compliments? The chef!) So much for the barnyard, how about the fields? If your mother, like mine, failed to bribe you with sufficient quarters to get you to eat your brussels sprouts, then you've consumed only about three acres of lettuce, a half-acre of string beans, and a divot or two of broccoli. You may have sown your wild oats, but you've never eaten them.

At 40, step onto the front porch of the farmhouse and survey the fat of the land off of which you've been living. Listen to the accusatory moos, bleats, oinks, and clucks of the livestock and poultry you've sheltered in that great barn protruding over your belt. If you continue eating like this, in another seven years you will have, in a manner of speaking, bought the farm.

After your first 40 years, it's time to plow up the back 40, as it were, and put in peas, beans, lentils, oats, and barley. When you've planted these seeds of countless boring monologues on the virtues of your diet, trade in your tractor for a Health Rider. Wouldn't you rather spend your 80th birthday on horseback in the wide open spaces of Wyoming than in a wheelchair in the narrow corridors of a nursing home? You'll be shouting "Yippee-yi-o!" in both places but they wouldn't have to medicate you for it in Wyoming.

Before putting the farm metaphor out to pasture, let me point out that you don't want to close the barn door after the horse is out by dieting and exercising *after* your heart attack. How pathetic! If your LDL cholesterol is high or if you've lost a young parent or sibling to heart disease, go vegan now and don't give me some mealy-mouthed excuse that roughage gives you gas.

Don't eat more than four eggs a week. I realize that telling you to monitor your egg consumption is like asking the fox to guard the henhouse. But if you don't, you'll be betraying yourself—fatally. You'll become your own Benedict Arnold. How do you think Eggs Benedict got its name?

You can have two drinks a day if you're a man, one drink if you're a woman, and eight drinks if you profit from the manufacture of cigarettes.

Your years of grazing are over. For each day of the rest of your life, you've got to impose a system of diet and exercise on yourself as if your mind were the warden of Devil's Island and your body a prisoner. A life sentence of bread and water and eight hours a day on the rock pile? Not quite. Start by joining the Devil's Island chapter of Weight Watchers. Punish your body in solitary confinement for twenty minutes three times a week on your Health Rider, NordicTrack, or Stairmaster.

Jane Fonda has taken to advertising the Health Rider on which I thankfully sit, now that she's put my knees out of commission with her workout tapes. Thirty years from now I expect her to be doing infomercials for the Stroke Rider, a square-tire nursing home wheelchair "that bulks your biceps for the race to the dining room." Ten years later, she'll be plugging the Jane Fonda Weight-Lifters Casket, fitted with "power-grip handles for your pallbearers to pump up their abs and pecs as they jerk and press you into the hearse."

Depending on your metabolism and your masochism, you can lose weight sooner or later on a low-fat, moderate carbohydrate, moderate protein diet, plus exercise. Until we can get our chubby hands on leptin, the fat-burning hormone, which will make us all as skinny as movie stars on 5000 calories a day, we've got to remember that fat has nine calories per gram, carbohydrate and protein only four.

Obesity and sagging muscles are what give old age a bad rep. Get lean and tough enough to look good for your body type and hold it right there. Don't waste your time suffering like an Egyptian slave over the great food pyramids. If you're overweight and still crave fat (which makes everything taste better), eat tiny portions and throw the rest away. Taste it and waste it! Gnash it and trash it! (Not recommended for those who can't stomach self-discipline or pithy slogans that rhyme.)

Take four small bites of a Quarter Pounder—one for each quadrant—slam dunk the rest and you're outta there. Good for you! You've chomped out maybe a Ninth of a Pounder—a hundred measly calories—containing just enough grease and salt to leave you with a queasy hint of satiety and a naughty twinge of guilt. (Rhyming slogan alert: After dinner, better a hint than a mint! Better a twinge than a binge!) Or eat the whole Quarter Pounder, without fries, and have only juice for the next meal. See if I care.

I keep a jar of fiery hot salsa in the fridge and scarf two tablespoons now and then for a no-cal heartburn that gives me the same feeling of molten glass slowly blown into a vase inside my belly as a high-cal heartburn. Treat yourself to little snacks of forbidden fruit or fat. Have an anchovy-stuffed olive, see if I care! Just one and you'll be up all night, thrashing off a hundred calories. Nosh a kosher dill pickle and feel just as bad as if you'd eaten the pastrami and rye that God decreed should accompany it.

Near the cash register in our local 7-Eleven, a worthy charity is dispensing bite-sized Snickers bars through a coin-operated container·

for only a quarter. This teensy bit of heaven comes fully wrapped. The world's best candy bar and maybe 40 calories, 50 tops. "Oh Callooh! Callay!" as Lewis Carroll cries in "Jabberwocky." I have one and sometimes two of these micro-Snickers. Again I quote: "One, two! One, two! And through and through the vorpal blade went snicker-snack!" (Did Carroll really say, "snicker-snack"?) By coincidence, my Swiss Army Knife has a vorpal blade designed to cut through and through each snicker snack, doubling my portions. What will those Swiss think of next—no-calorie holes in cheese?

Use all the salt you want unless you have high blood pressure or heart failure. Otherwise, salt to taste! In ancient times, armies went to war for salt. New restaurants with gorgeous interiors, impeccable service, and seductive menus go out of business in six months, leaving their owners and chefs dumbfounded. Why? Because they undersalted their food. They were so fearful of turning off the health nuts that they turned off the *fressers*. Dig into the foundation of any enduringly successful restaurant and you'll come upon a pillar of salt and a slab of grease.

Giving up grease is tough enough. Giving up grease and salt will only send you out at three in the morning to the nearest 7-Eleven, where you'll pull a gun and shout, "Four jumbo chili cheese dogs in 30 seconds or you're dead meat!"

If you've been able to give up the chili cheese dog or the Beef Wellington in favor of the Rock Cornish Game Hen (or the Doc Ornish game plan), reward yourself. For each fortnight during the next 40 years, schedule a 4000 calorie blow-out at an enduringly successful restaurant. This amounts to a thousand and one nights in the Fat City Diner, the last feast being your 80th birthday bash.

By your 41st birthday, when you've toned and semi-starved yourself to what you looked and felt like at 23, you can maintain your weight and your health if you eat strictly out of a Mediterranean cookbook and up your time on the Health Rider to 16 hours a day. Do you have a problem with that?

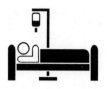

RULE 22:

Drive a Full-Sized American Car

Managed care is positively boring in its emphasis on preventive health measures. So am I. What could be more protective of our fragile bodies—crumple zones everywhere!—than belting up in a car as big as the Ritz?

I drive a four-year-old Lincoln Town Car, the only full-sized American car in the People's Republic of Berkeley. I'm embarrassed to give you its exact measurements, but a whitish spot that resembles a rather large bird dropping on its left front fender is actually a Hyundai.

As we drive bumper to bumper into the millennium, the race will not be won by the little, the shifty, and the swift, but by the big, the automatic, and the sluggish. There is no longer any room for us to cut in front of our opposition: we must roll over them. In sheer size, my Lincoln Town Car does not take a back seat to any passenger vehicle, with the possible exception of the Cadillac Fleetwood Brougham, which became extinct in Berkeley two years ago when the last one tried to ram a Lincoln Town Car. At intersections, I don't even yield to buses (*AC Transit v. London,* 1976, 1983, 1994).

The next time you take the DMV driver's test and you come to the multiple-choice question about who at an intersection has the right of way, write in "Lincoln Town Car" and you'll be moved to the head of the line to have your picture taken, followed by your fingerprints, and permission to make one phone call.

There is no question that my Town Car commands respect. Whenever I drive along Berkeley's San Pablo Boulevard between Dwight Way and Woolsey, drug dealers who normally slouch in doorways stride to the curb, snap to attention, realize it's only me, and slouch back to their doorways.

Above all, I believe in the supremacy of the full-sized American car, despite the fact that *Road & Track* voted the Bittburg 793i "Car of the Year." My Lincoln may have a frequency-of-repair record that rated a cover story in last month's issue of *Towed & Rack*, but let me hasten to point out that its frequent appearances in body shops are solely my fault and not that of the Ford Motor Company, where "Quality is Job One." My motto is "Collision Insurance is Job One."

Owners of body shops dance in the streets after they hand me their appraisal of damage costs. My car has driven several body shop owners to early retirement in Palm Springs. The only way I was able to get an auto insurance company to stay with me through the years was to marry one of its agents. Ours is the only marriage contract that guarantees full replacement of all damaged body parts (exclusive of coupling assembly and emissions control systems).

The inside of my Lincoln Town Car resembles a lawyer's office. The plush beige carpeting and simulated-wood paneling give off the aura of confident litigiousness so essential to a driver's peace of mind in the 90s.

Of course, the major virtue of my full-sized American car is armor plating. I can drive up a narrow, twisting road in the Berkeley hills and suddenly confront a six-door Bittburg bearing down on me and BAM, there goes the Bittburg over an embankment and into a free fall of 200 feet. On its way down it shows off its famous acceleration from zero to 60 in eight seconds. I will say to the credit of the oft-maligned Bittburg drivers, that they have uniformly saluted me during their rapid descent in the chivalrous manner of stricken Fokker pilots during WW I dog fights.

I don't want to give the impression that I go out of my way to inflict damage on tailgating, signal-jumping, road-hogging cars of smaller size, built in countries that opposed us in World War II. I have come to believe that my Lincoln Town Car collides with lesser vehicles in accordance with the gravitational principle that a full-sized mass attracts a mid-sized one. If you suggest I tell that to the judge, let me assure you I have.

RULE 23:

Write Your Own Medical Journal and Make Sure Your Doctor Subscribes to It

Managed Care devours time. You've got to catch your doctor on the run. Wrestle him into undistracted attention and pummel him with your complaints. He hasn't got time to listen to you grope for details. If you want to survive Managed Care, learn to write succinct, accurate notes to your doctor. If done well, these notes can help your doctor save your life or, at least, refill your Valium prescription.

Herewith is an example of the kind of note I like to see. It's written by one of my patients, Mr. Robert Houlehan, a 68-year-old retired kindergarten teacher, saxophonist, jazz DJ, *bon vivant*, wine buff, and Francophile. His love of food and wine often conflicts with a fierce desire to keep fit enough to indulge his appetites. He has graciously consented to let me print one of his informative, lively notes to me, his doctor, and to discuss his case.

As I walk into the exam room, this large, happy man with a ruddy face and booming voice sits regally on an armchair in the corner. On the lapel of his black suit are jewel-like medallions of the various wine and gourmet societies to which he ardently belongs, along with a small, silver saxophone pin. He wears these like military decorations. On the countertop against the wall, he has ceremoniously placed a bottle of excellent Sonoma County wine that acts as a paperweight for his medical note *du jour.*

August 10, 1995

THE STATE OF ROBERT V. HOULEHAN
(Just call him "Slim.")

Weight—223, down 20 pounds in three months!

Labors of Health—walking 30 minutes (briskly) three times a week. Swimming 45 minutes (slowly) twice a week. Eating 400 calories (instantly) three times a day.

Prescription Drugs—Allopurinol 300 mg. at bedtime, Zantac 150 mg. twice daily, Zestril 10 mg. in a.m., Lopid 600 mg. twice daily, Lopressor 50 mg. in a.m., Proscar 5 mg. in a.m., Baby aspirin one in a.m., Fioricet up to 4 times a day for headache, Temazepam 15 mg. at bedtime.

Problems—left shoulder aches, ears plugged with wax. Headaches. Slight stomach pain (peptic ulcer?).

Travel—to Spain and Morocco end of April. Shots?

Overall Condition—fine as wine in the summertime!

Wine—I almost never recommend a port not made in Portugal. However, a few small California wineries produce limited amounts of California port of excellent quality. This is one. Enjoy!

L.W. Morris 1983 Vintage
Sonoma County
Old Vines Hill

P.S. I suggest this be served at a slightly chilled temperature (56°).

In a few, well-chosen words on his Macintosh, Mr. Houlehan has filled me in on his symptoms, health habits, current medications, and the contents of the fine bottle of wine he brings me each visit. Besides his description of the port, the most important part of his document is the up-to-date list of his many medications used to treat his various conditions: gout (Allopurinol); hypertension (Lopressor); high triglycerides plus low HDL cholesterol (Lopid); gastritis (Zantac) and enlarged prostate (Proscar), to name more than a few.

With a glance at his note, I can tell if I've inadvertently prescribed duplicate medications or conflicting ones. When I see a patient who takes the trouble to write down his drugs, I'm confident that he's taking the trouble to use them as directed.

I stand accused of inflicting polypharmacy on the rotund body of Robert V. Houlehan. Most of the drugs I prescribe for him treat the consequences of his gourmandizing: hypertension, high triglycerides, gout, and gastritis. If I had absolute power to force him to give up wining and dining in the world's best restaurants, he could throw almost all his medications away. Three months later, the message he'd write would not be one of his jovial, state-of-the-health-bulletins, but a suicide note. I prefer he remain a pill-popping, fun-loving, viable gourmand than a fit, lean, and dead health nut.

My prescription for Mr. Houlehan is eat, drink, and be merry, diet between three-star restaurants, exercise daily, and take your pills with a large glass of water and my apologies.

Mr. Houlehan may be a retired teacher, but he hasn't stopped instructing me about his health, his travels, and his wine. For taking such terrific care of himself and his doctor, Managed Care thanks him and so do I.

Vive le Houlehan!

RULE 24:

Meditate to Survive the Thousand Deaths of Daily Living

I die 31 deaths just waiting in line at Baskin-Robbins. If the ice cream doesn't kill me some day, the customers in front of me will. Nothing induces a transient ischemic attack in me more readily than listening to the obese customer in tight shorts six places down the line assault the clerk with endless revisions of his order:

"Instead of a double scoop of pralines and cream, make that a single scoop of chocolate fudge, oh, and gimme two scoops of banana walnut with hot fudge topping, hold the nuts and cherries, but lots of whipped cream and, oh, can you change that scoop of chocolate fudge back to one of pralines and cream and one of peanut butter fudge? Wait! I want them on a sugar cone and come on, that's not a full scoop, mister, dig in...."

In the darkroom of my imagination I develop a picture of this customer's brain: a junior-sized scoop of smooth, unconvoluted vanilla ice cream.

It's too bad that rubbing out a customer inside a United States Post Office is a Federal offense. If looks could kill, I'd be sorely tempted to throw myself on the mercy of a court for staring daggers at the skinny back of that young man with a robin's-egg-blue ponytail and one hip cocked lazily, standing immobile at the counter for the past 24 minutes. (Or is he dead already?)

I find similar permanent fixtures appearing at the heads of lines in supermarkets, car rental agencies, and movie theaters. I believe these stationary objects should be rounded up and sold as lawn ornaments before they completely stop Western Civilization in its tracks.

The cumulative stresses of queuing up would be more than I could bear if I hadn't discovered the wonders of meditation. I learned to meditate by purchasing a $120 mantra from a used karma lot in 1963. Today, I could get over $3,000 for my vintage '63 mantra, but I wouldn't trade it in for a classic, off-road ashram with floor mats and a million oms on its odometer. Meditation has saved not only my sanity but also the lives of countless patrons of Baskin-Robbins and the post office.

For submitting a note from your guru that you meditate regularly, Managed Care should issue you a discount on your premium. In recent years, I've recommended to my patients a western spin-off of transcendental meditation called "The Relaxation Response." Dr. Herbert Benson of Harvard has westernized the TM technique by having his patients sit comfortably on a chair or sofa in the couch-potato—as opposed to the lotus—position, breathe in and out through their nose and say the word "one" as they exhale (Benson, Herbert, *The Relaxation Response.* New York: Avon Books, 1976).

I've been meditating 15 minutes each morning for more than thirty years in the hushed lobby of Berkeley's swank Claremont Hotel near my office. As a result, I've accumulated a great measure of inner peace and spirtual strength, not to mention over $41,000 in coins extracted from the sofa cushions.

Under Managed Care, you will have to wait longer than ever to see your doctor. What better way to kill time in the waiting room than to meditate? After all, meditation rivals medication in lowering your blood pressure, pulse rate, respirations per minute, and circulating adrenalin. After meditating and accumulating gas for two hours in my waiting room, my patients levitate an average of four inches off the chair. They are then gently airlifted by Tammie, my nurse of serene visage, to a cubicle inside my office. There they languidly disrobe, then wait just 15 minutes more while I meditate to recover from my last patient.

RULE 25:

Know When to Call Your Doctor

Under Managed Care, patients often hate to bother their overworked doctor. Through your HMO's capitation plan, your employer has already paid your doctor for your body whether he sees it or not. Why burden the poor guy with your hypochondriacal problems when he already has his hands full seeing real patients? In this new age of medicine, it behooves you to know when it's time to "get real," as the teenagers say. I will now teach you when it's appropriate to demand of Her Royal Majesty, your doctor's secretary, that you be worked into his busy schedule the same day.

It's amazing to me how considerate my patients are. They're reluctant to burden me with their trivial complaints. From such niceness a patient could die. "Doc, I hate to take up your time, but for the past week I've been getting this funny little feeling in the center of my chest whenever I take a walk. It's not even a pain, just a little stuffiness. I don't even know why I'm bothering you."

The patient's next words are, "But you can't put me in the hospital now! My car's parked in your garage downstairs!" This patient has just described new-onset angina pectoris, a prelude to an often-fatal heart attack and a near-fatal parking fee.

Two weeks later, he's showing off his chest scar from the triple-bypass surgery. If he had been any nicer to me, his buddies at the office would be admiring not the beauty of his scar, but how terrific his nattily attired body looked during the memorial service. Ask any embalmer: coronaries make the prettiest corpses.

As a rule, it takes women 10 to 20 years longer than men to have their heart attacks, but when they do, they're not as likely as men to survive them. A woman's heart pain is more apt to occur at rest than a man's. Last year, a female patient of mine failed to report her vague chest pains to me because she was having a bad hair day and Raoul had kindly squeezed her into his busy schedule. Fortunately, when she complained of having a chest pain in his chair, Raoul persuaded her to call me from his salon. He ended up doing her hair in the coronary care unit three days after her successful bypass surgery. He assured her that he would have been willing to do her at the mortuary, but wasn't sure the embalmer would permit him to do a permanent.

In contrast to those who drop dead from heart attacks, stroke victims require quite a little facial and limb manipulation before they can be properly laid out. These are people who were too considerate of their doctor's precious time to have him check their blood pressure and cholesterol or to bother telling him, "For a few minutes this morning, my right arm and leg got a little weak and my wife said I slurred my words. Then I felt fine." This is the classic description of a transient ischemic attack (TIA), a harbinger of a stroke.

If given a 24-hour handicap, a doctor can often save a patient's life if he learns about those TIAs shortly after they occur. Sometimes a doctor can listen to a patient's neck with his stethoscope and detect signs of an easily removable fatty deposit in a carotid artery. A suspicion of carotid narrowing can be confirmed by a painless ultrasound scan of the neck. In a relatively simple and safe operation, a vascular surgeon can scoop out the glob of fat, dramatically preventing a stroke. Lesson: Bare your soul and your neck to your doctor.

Most people die of strokes and heart attacks between 4:00 and 10:00 A.M. In other words, they took the two aspirin and failed to call their doctor in the morning. If you wake up alive at 7:00 A.M., dress, shower, and drive to the office very slowly. Then wait until after 10:00 A.M. to have your first cigarette, which will not likely kill you for at least another 18 hours.

You don't have to be reminded to call your doctor when you suffer severe dizziness at rest or on standing. The odd thing is, if you recover fully by the time you arrive at his office, there's very little for him to do as a rule, but examine you and pronounce you healthy.

The most common type of dizziness is vertigo—a loss of balance or a spinning sensation. Vertigo is a miserable thing to experience, but it's rarely symptomatic of a stroke. Instead, it's a disturbance of the organ of balance located deep within the bone behind your ear, just shy of your brain. The only really effective treatment for vertigo is time, which is dispensed more liberally in a doctor's waiting room than in his office. Often as not, by the time my receptionist ushers you in, your vertigo is cured.

A man who gets overwhelmingly sleepy in the afternoon should drink a cup of black coffee and quickly call his doctor for an appointment before he nods off again. He may be suffering from sleep apnea, seen mostly in overweight men who drink and snore. Apnea means an absence of breathing and that's what this fat man suffers if he boozes before he snoozes. The soft tissues in the back of his throat grow slack from fatigue and bourbon, resulting in either partial blockage of breathing (snoring) or complete blockage (apnea).

Each of these frequent spells of apnea can last over a minute, resulting in no oxygen getting to his brain, until he takes his next deep breath. Throughout the night, his oxygen-starved brain is frequently startled to partial wakefulness, depriving him of essential deep sleep. In the morning, if his apnea has not killed him with a stroke or heart attack, he's exhausted, as is his bed partner from his window-rattling snores and his suspenseful breath-holding.

The cure for the apneic partner is dieting, teetotaling, sleeping on his side and, failing that, wearing a light, positive-pressure oxygen mask to bed. At times, submitting to a simple operation to remove some of the redundant tissue in the back of his throat will allow him to give up the mask and sleep like a baby, eat like a hog, and drink like a fish. The definitive cure for his bed partner is divorce or a separate bedroom.

If we're lucky, strokes and heart attacks give us advance notice, and if we're smart, we call our doctor for help pronto. Cancer is another matter. There are few distant early warning signs of cancer. One is the appearance of a smoking white cylinder protruding from your mouth. If you can't remove it permanently, see your doctor who will perform an emergency Camelectomy before your very eyes.

If you wait for a change in bowel habits or weight loss to have yourself checked out for colorectal cancer, you're too late. If, starting at age 50, you insist on having a sigmoidoscopy or barium enema every five years to look for pre-cancerous polyps, you'll end up 30 years later with the most envied rectum in the nursing home. (You wouldn't be there, of course, if you'd remembered to take your blood pressure pills.)

To paraphrase Dr. Morris A. Samuels of Harvard, if you're worried about having Alzheimer's disease and remember to call your doctor about it, forget it—you don't have Alzheimer's. If you forget to call your doctor about it, you've got Alzheimer's, but you won't know it, so why worry? ("Neurological Update," *Audio-Digest Internal Medicine,* Vol. 42, March 1995)

Most memory loss that we suffer after age 50 is due to what's called benign senescent forgetfulness—all of us have it or will get it—and if you can remember to recite that diagnosis whenever you grope for a word, you don't have Alzheimer's disease. If you can't remember benign senescent forgetfulness, call Dr. Samuels.

Other incentives to speed-dial your doctor are:

the appearance of red or blackened blood in the stool

blood in the urine (seldom proves serious)

blood with ejaculation (never proves serious)

getting up more than twice each night to urinate

burning pain on urination

abdominal pain lasting more than an hour

temperature above 103°F

cough with yellow, green, or bloody sputum

"crowing" respiration during a throat infection

sharp chest pain whenever you inhale

severe wheezing

increased frequency and severity of headaches

headache and stiff neck with or without fever

sudden dimming or loss of vision in one eye even if it lasts for a short time

excruciating back pain not relieved by lying down

a red swollen joint

diarrhea or vomiting to the point of lightheadedness

vomiting what looks like coffee grounds (may be blood or Sanka)

diarrhea of any severity for more than three weeks

discovery of a breast lump or a pitch-black mole

a swollen, warm, tender leg (may be phlebitis)

irregular and/or rapid heart beat (more than 100 beats per minute at rest)

severe shortness of breath at rest (may indicate heart attack, blood clots in lungs, or just anxiety)

a day or more of marked thirst, hunger, weakness, and passing large amounts of urine (diagnostic of diabetes or Yom Kippur)

If you suffer from none of the above, call your travel agent and book a Caribbean cruise. If you hear of an opening for a ship's surgeon, call me at once.

RULE 26:

Don't Wait for the Embalmer to Take 10 Years off Your Age

Managed Care does not recognize cosmetic surgery. What did you expect from a faceless organization? Pity the last survivors of fee-for-service: the brow-lifters, fat-suckers, and tummy-tuckers. How can these docs make ends meet out there alone? Very well, it seems. I know of one nose-bobbing butt-lifter, who, out of embarrassment, had his Rolls Royce customized to resemble an Oldsmobile Cutlass.

Father Time grabs us first by the throat. The unsightly, loose chicken skin of the neck first appears—seemingly overnight—at about age 50. A woman can cope with this by ignoring it, scarving it, or lifting it. The last maneuver requires the help of a plastic surgeon, that restorer of youth to the rich and famous.

A man sometimes copes with his chicken neck by seeing if he can attract a chick. Failing that, he deals with his sagging neck by ignoring it, cravating it, bearding it, or lifting it. At 50, men aren't nearly as eager as women to bare their face or neck to the knife of a cosmetic surgeon. Perhaps men are more prone than women to be put off by the uncommon but horrific risks of discomfort, deformity, and death from plastic surgery. After all, as George Orwell pointed out admiringly, "At fifty, a man gets the face he deserves." Our society often labels a man handsome after he undergoes tissue changes that are deemed unattractive in a woman.

Then the cheeks droop, the lips wrinkle, the eyelids bag, the abdomen sags, the butt drags, and the chicken neck turns turkeyish. Finally, liver spots appear on the forehead and temples like coffee stains on a roughly sketched caricature of a once-attractive face. Mayday!

Men start appearing sheepishly alongside women in the beige and gold Louis XIV waiting rooms of celebrity surgeons.

It's unfortunate that in our country only the rich can afford cosmetic surgery, which, if performed well, takes years off the appearance of whatever the surgeon works on: your face (10 years), abdomen (12 years), buttocks (14 years), and breasts (20 years). Numerous studies have shown that good-looking people are perceived as more popular, smarter, and better at dealing with other people (*Developmental Psychology*, May 1995). None but the most affluent can afford the best revenge—living well—and the second-best revenge—looking good.

Brazil is light-years ahead of us in plastic surgery. You don't think for a minute that all those beautiful faces and bodies on the beaches of Rio are a fluke of nature? That sucking sound you hear south of the border is not the drain of American jobs as Ross Perot insists, but rather the 13 thousand liposuctions performed daily in Rio. Brazil has more plastic surgeons per balding and wrinkled capita than any country in the world.

According to my friend Gerald the proctologist, you can have liposuction right on the beach at Ipenema in a cabaña. You can lie back on a chaise lounge and sip a piña colada through a straw while your *médico cosmetico* sucks out your saddle bags with a trochar and dune-buggy hearses patrol the beach outside for the occasional hasty burial at sea. Gerald tends toward hyperbole, but I must say that since flying back from Rio, he looks at least 14 years younger from the rear when he bends down to pick up a golf ball at his country club. He says he had to stand up in first class during the entire return flight.

Some years back, the Oakland School District offered its teachers possibly the only health plan in America that included elective cosmetic surgery. (I am not making this up.) For five years, the students looked to their teachers for the three R's: reading, writing, and rhinoplasty. The faculty was on sick leave so often that the brighter students' grades went from A to D while their teachers' bra sizes did the same. An outraged and impoverished citizenry finally persuaded the school district that the money would be better spent raising students' SATs than teachers' derrières.

If our HMOs persist in refusing to cover cosmetic surgery, then I say the government should step in. A face-lift for every citizen should be grandfathered into the Contract with America. Clearly, in this age of downsizing, massive layoffs, Managed Care, and drive-by shootings, it's difficult for Americans to keep their chins up, maintain stiff upper lips, breast the turbulent seas of change, and put their noses to the grindstone without surgical assistance.

We may never be the healthiest or smartest nation in the world, but I see no reason why we can't be the best looking. Let's give the sagging face of our nation a much-needed lift, and show the world that we are, indeed, America the Beautiful!

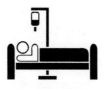

RULE 27:

Know When to Fire Your Doctor

Under Managed Care, you have a limited choice of who's going to be your primary care physician but you needn't feel stuck with your first choice. You can always return the unused portion of your doctor to your HMO and hope you'll have better luck with his generic equivalent.

From having lost my share of unhappy patients and having won a passel of other doctors' angry ones, I think I can advise you to fire your doctor when he or she:

1. *Fails to return phone calls.* More medicine is transacted by telephone than I care to admit. Although no substitute for seeing the doctor in person, the telephone is a powerful tool of medical communication. There's no excuse for a doctor's not returning your phone call the same day you make it, unless you tell his receptionist it's okay for him to call you tomorrow.

If the call is not urgent, forgive your doctor's delay in returning the call but do not tolerate silence as his ultimate response. If you're at a difficult phone or can't wait to be called later, ask that the doctor step out of the restroom and pick up the phone now. If you've waited in vain for a response for more than two hours, call him back.

Through the years, when I've been on night call for other doctors, I've been astonished at how often their patients apologize for calling me because their own doctor had failed to return their call earlier in the day. If your doctor continues to snub you, call his secretary and have her tell him you're finding another doctor and if he has any questions, not to call you.

2. *Refuses to see you ASAP.* If you have a bad cough or other acute misery and want to see your doctor, there's no excuse for not being seen the same day or, if it can wait, the next day. Again, I can't believe my ears when former patients of other doctors tell me they

were given an appointment three weeks hence for an abdominal pain! If you're acutely ill, ask the receptionist if she can possibly fit you into today's schedule. If she says, "No," ask her boss to fit you in.

I myself encourage these "work-in" patients. First of all, it's medically necessary that they be examined the same day. Secondly, they're very grateful for being seen so promptly and therefore careful not to take more time than necessary. Finally, they'll understand during a future, routine appointment that I might be running late due to spending extra time with an acutely ill patient, as I had with them.

3. *Never in the office.* Some doctors spend a lot of their energy absenting themselves from the office. They're at the hospital, they're "en route," they're attending a meeting in Brussels, they're giving expert testimony in court, they're sick in bed, or they're on their fourth vacation in six months. One of your doctor's long-suffering partners ends up seeing you reluctantly. Your own doctor is a name on the door and a body in the Bahamas.

Sometimes your doctor may be technically in the office, but his mind may be elsewhere. If your doctor is playing hooky, ask your HMO for the name of another primary care physician, preferably one who is in his office at least four and a half days a week, eleven months a year, and is "out-to-lunch" only during the lunch hour.

4. *Keeps you waiting endlessly.* I usually ask my scheduled patients to bear with me during office hours because of unscheduled delays and interruptions. But if your own schedule is as busy or busier than your doctor's and if he consistently keeps you waiting for more than an hour, ask if he can possibly see you sooner or you'll have to find another doctor. Take it from me, if you express your displeasure in these terms, at your next visit a nurse will show you to an exam room with the élan of a maître d' escorting Donald Trump to a power table at Lutece.

Of course, you'll be stranded for the next hour lying on a table before Dr. Generic or one of his clones can see you. Did you expect a shorter wait under Managed Care than you suffered under fee-for-service? Hah! At least under fee-for-service, your doctor could afford to heat the office and provide you with a commodious, cloth gown. With Managed Care, you must sit shivering on the exam table in a paper tee shirt while the secretary sees if your HMO will approve a referral to a urologist. A urologist? Now calm down. A clerical error must have been made in the front office. I, Oscar London, M.D., W.B.D, would gladly help you, but I'm not assigned to this table.

RULE 28:

Only Bad Doctors Advertise

In my not-so-humble opinion, advertising is the last refuge of the medical scoundrel. Perhaps I am putting that too strongly. Let me just say that doctors who advertise are an embarrassment to those of us who don't. Managed Care has encouraged certain doctors or groups of doctors to advertise. The profit motive of the care managers has proved contagious to the care givers. Nothing on television makes me cringe more acutely than the sight of a powerfully built young man wearing a white coat and a beatific smile gazing warmly into the eye of the camera while a voice-over proclaims:

"At Infirminente, orthopedic surgeon and cabinet maker Dr. Bradley Marvel talks about his last patient.

DR. MARVEL: I told this elderly gentleman that he needed to have his right hip replaced and he asked me if I could build a drawer in the prosthesis so he could store some of his smaller valuables and I said, 'Sure, why not'?

VOICE-OVER: At Infirminente, when our patients speak, we listen."

In the past five years, I've been saddened to see how many physicians have flouted a 100-year-old tradition of American medicine that frowned on advertising. Judging from the proliferation of ads by doctors who perform hair transplants and penile enhancements, you might get the erroneous impression that baldness and genital size were major concerns in the male population. Nothing could be further from the truth. Just ask the man in the street, as I did, what he desires most in life. "A roof over my head," is the universal answer of these male street people.

To illustrate my bias against aggressive self-promotion by Managed Care groups, hospitals, and individual doctors, let me cite the case history of Dr. Melvin I. Weintraub, a middle-aged cardiologist in my community. Two years ago, he suffered an alarming loss of patients as a result of a sudden flood of young heart specialists into a new building down the block. After much soul-searching and book-keeping, Dr. Weintraub decided to advertise. The first ad, if it can be called that, was simply the use of bold-face type in the Yellow Pages:

Melvin I. Weintraub, M.D., Inc.

Cardiologist

By Appointment Only (415) 555-1241

When the anticipated storming of his office by hordes of new patients failed to occur, Dr. Weintraub took the next step, a one-by-two-inch print ad in five San Francisco Bay Area weeklies:

Melvin I. Weintraub, M.D., Inc., Cardiologist

"The Patients' Choice" Validated Parking

VISA and MasterCard Accepted

(415) 555-1241

For two weeks his phone rang off the hook. Then, like a defrosting windshield, his appointment book developed large clear spaces. In desperation, he hired a photographer who took a color portrait of Dr. Weintraub seated at his desk, staring compassionately (his colleagues would say beseechingly) into the camera. Slightly soft-focused on the wall just behind him glowed his diploma from a prestigious New England medical school.

Under orders from Dr. Weintraub, the photographer touched up the 54-year-old doctor's head, air-brushing in clumps of hair that Weintraub had lost in the line of duty, removing a wart here, adding a dimple there, inking out most of the gray at his temples, but leaving a small, distinguished streak (unfortunately on only one side). The completed picture was a slightly flawed masterpiece that appeared for 15 seconds on a cable TV channel specializing in art films. A voice-over proclaimed:

"Does your doctor's face get a faraway look while he's listening to your heart? He's probably thinking of his golf game or he's so deaf he might as well be pressing his stethoscope to a chest of drawers! Dr. Melvin I. Weintraub, a fellow of the American College of Cardiology, has the ears of a bat and has never picked up a golf club in his life. You'll never see a faraway look on his face. As reassurance that he's not being distracted, Dr. Weintraub will often burst into tears while listening to a patient's heart.

"This week only, Dr. Weintraub is offering a complimentary blood pressure reading to the first 20 patients who call this toll free number: 1-800-555-6753. Operators are standing by."

Actually, only Mrs. Gertrude Weintraub, Melvin's mother, was standing by. The incredible response to the TV ad was reminiscent of the advance ticket sales to *Phantom of the Opera*. After more than two decades, Dr. Weintraub's practice finally took off.

The group of young hot-shot cardiologists down the block retaliated the next week with a TV spot in which the camera panned over a cemetery for a few seconds, and then over a golf course. A voice-over proclaimed:

"Dr. Melvin Weintraub's older patients spend every Wednesday afternoon surrounded by trees and grass... (shot of cemetery)

"So do ours... (shot of golf course)

"This has been a public service message brought to you by the Lakeside Cardiology Group."

The brouhaha resulting from the barrage of competitive advertising resulted in land-office business for both Dr. Weintraub and the Lakeside Cardiology Group.

Three months ago, Mrs. H., my least favorite patient, called my office for the third time in a week to talk to me. In a voice that caused small fractures to appear in the lenses of my reading glasses, she complained that I never listened to her and that she still had terrible chest pains. Since nothing I gave her worked; why should her HMO have to foot the bill?

"In what part of your foot are these pains?" I asked.

"Not my foot, my chest! You never listen!"

"Mrs H.," I said, "I've got an idea. Let me refer you to a cardiologist, Dr. Melvin I. Weintraub, for a consultation."

"Oh yeah," said Mrs. H., her voice softening to a roar. "I saw him on television. Now there's a man who looks like a doctor!"

Suddenly experiencing mild vertigo, I gave her Dr. Weintraub's toll-free number.

A week later, our medical community was shocked to learn that Dr. Melvin I. Weintraub had dropped dead in his office shortly after examining a female patient. By inflicting Mrs. H. on Dr. Weintraub I had merely wanted to express my disapproval of doctors who advertise. I had not meant to kill him.

Under Managed Care, I am finding it increasingly difficult to refer patients to specialists and when I succeed, look what happens.

RULE 29:

Try Not to Be an "Interesting Case"

As an internist in private practice, the last thing I want to see is an "interesting case." By definition (mine), an interesting case is a very sick patient without a diagnosis. It's the medical equivalent of an unsolved crime. In a detective novel, the aggrieved party hires a "private eye" (private investigator) to solve the crime. In medicine, the patient with a mysterious illness also turns to a "private eye" (private internist) to make the diagnosis.

The most interesting case I've had in more than three decades of practicing internal medicine began conventionally enough about four years ago. A strapping young man of 27, whom I will call Michael, was struck in the abdomen by his 10-year-old nephew during an impromptu round of boxing at a family picnic. As Michael recalled, the blow caused a very uncomfortable lower abdominal pain that after a few hours subsided into a dull ache. When the ache did not go away after two weeks, Michael consulted me.

His past medical history was "unremarkable," a medical buzzword sometimes indicating that the doctor has not spent enough time talking to the patient or his family. Michael's physical examination revealed mild, lower abdominal tenderness. I noted that his legs seemed slightly swollen and that a small varicose vein bulged beneath the skin of his right upper thigh. Otherwise, he resembled Jack Armstrong, the All-American Boy. I concluded that I didn't know the exact cause of his abdominal pain and could only guess at about twelve possibilities. Michael was beginning to resemble an "interesting case."

To reduce the possibilities, I put Michael through a series of blood tests and X-ray examinations, culminating in a CAT scan of his abdomen. The blood tests and routine abdominal X-rays were all normal, but his CAT scan revealed a shocker. Two large, oval masses sat inside his pelvis like a pair of ostrich eggs. Each measured five to six inches in diameter and lay deep within the pelvic cavity, behind the pubic bone. Therefore, they could not be felt on physical exam. (Chalk up another diagnostic triumph to the CAT scan, a high-tech image frequently deemed "not cost-effective" by an HMO.) The diagnostic possibilities, in my mind, had tragically narrowed to cancer of the lymph nodes.

I kept Michael and his family abreast of all test results and informed them that the large masses seen in his pelvis on the CAT scan looked like cancer, but hastened to add that, until a surgical biopsy gave us a piece of tissue to put under a microscope, I could not be sure of the diagnosis. Privately, I was certain it was cancer, but technically I was correct in pointing out that a biopsy was essential to a precise diagnosis in this case. After I unloaded my diagnostic thoughts on Michael, the usually relaxed expression on his tanned, handsome face suddenly froze into a pale, haunted look.

I asked a surgeon to examine Michael. Because of the baffling (i.e., "interesting") features of the case, the surgeon, Dr. Robert Gaynor, recommended an exploratory abdominal operation to afford a direct look at the ominous masses. Dr. Gaynor was also convinced that the large lumps would turn out to be malignant. He, too, was struck by Michael's swollen legs and postulated that the tumors were pressing on his pelvic veins, causing a damming of upward blood flow from his leg veins below.

Michael's case became even more interesting at surgery. The pelvic masses, exposed by Dr. Gaynor's incision, turned out to be two enormous blood clots encased in a thin shell of scar tissue. They were masses consisting of old blood, not cancer!

His young nephew's punch to Michael's midsection had evidently been more powerful than Michael was willing to admit: the blow had caused considerable bleeding inside his abdomen. The consolidation of the blood into clots and their partial scarring were natural reactions of Michael's body to an internal hemorrhage. The surgeon carefully checked Michael's spleen, a frequent source of traumatic bleeding inside the abdomen. The spleen was normal. Dr. Gaynor deftly excised the two blood clots, thereby apparently removing all obstruction to the venous flow. He closed his incision with the elation so frequently enjoyed by surgeons who believe they have cured the patient with their operation.

The rejoicing shared by Michael, his family, and physicians was tempered somewhat when, a week after surgery, Michael's legs had not lost their swelling, contrary to what we had predicted after the removal of the pelvic masses. In fact, if anything, his legs were more swollen than before surgery. A repeat CAT scan showed no more blood clots in his pelvis. Interesting.

One of the most dreaded complications of any major surgery is postoperative thrombophlebitis, the formation of blood clots within the veins of the pelvis or legs. These clots might break off into clumps called emboli, shoot up through the abdominal veins toward the chest, and lodge fatally inside the lungs. Whereas Michael's surgery revealed that he had formed blood clots outside his pelvic veins, his postoperative leg swelling suggested that he had now formed blood clots inside them.

The emotional roller coaster all of us were on took another sickening dip when dye was injected into Michael's leg veins, and X-rays revealed that not only were several deep veins in his thighs totally blocked, but his vena cava, the main vein in his abdomen, was choked shut four inches above its origin. His vena cava, which normally routes blood from his legs through his abdomen up to the right side of his heart, suddenly came to a dead end. Very interesting.

The presence of venous obstruction is a medical emergency requiring intravenous anticoagulants to prevent further clotting and the possible breaking off of deadly emboli. The ball was now in the internist's court. I accordingly ordered intravenous heparin with a prayer that in this young man who had so recently bled, the anticoagulant would not promote another major hemorrhage.

With Michael's consent, Dr. Gaynor and I called in Dr. David Levine (since deceased), a professor of hematology at U.C. San Francisco Medical School across the bay. Dr. Levine was as brilliant as he was bald and there wasn't a single hair on his scalp. He was a doctor's doctor, a profoundly knowledgeable and creative thinker—a magic diagnostician. Dr. Levine spent two hours questioning Michael and his mother about his past and present medical problems, and another hour examining him.

During the course of his questioning, Dr. Levine asked Michael's mother if her son had been jaundiced at birth, that is, was he a "yellow baby." His mother nodded, "Yes," and then recalled he had received an exchange transfusion "through a vein in his right leg" shortly after birth. The dignified Dr. Levine uncharacteristically leaped to his feet at that moment and punched the air in front of him once. The hematologist had his diagnosis.

Dr. Levine's question about Michael's having been jaundiced at birth was simply brilliant. I should have asked it of Michael and his parents when I first examined him. It was a question a medical student might ask more readily than a seasoned physician. Out of ignorance, a medical student asks every question in the book; out of "experience," a veteran doctor asks fewer but presumably more pointed questions. Dr. Levine's questions were more numerous than a medical student's and, at the same time, more pointed than mine.

When Michael's mother nodded, "Yes," the multi-tiered diagnosis suddenly crystallized:

1. The thin tube (or catheter) through which the exchange transfusion was given to baby Michael had been inserted into his right femoral (or leg) vein, then threaded up into his vena cava, where the irritation of the catheter provoked a massive inflammation and blood clot (thrombophlebitis).

2. The thrombophlebitis led to the formation of obstructing scar tissue, which caused a permanent blockage of his vena cava.

3. The blocked vena cava resulted in a lifelong, marked increase of blood pressure within the veins below his vena cava, namely, the veins in his pelvis and legs. The venous blood from his legs and pelvis ran up against this obstruction and backed up, causing increased pressure in these blood vessels. This impeded blood flow eventually made its way to the heart through small, "collateral" veins around the blocked vena cava.

4. His nephew's punch below the belt abruptly increased further the pressure within his already distended pelvic veins, causing a hemorrhagic blowout and the resulting two huge blood clots.

5. Compression from the pelvic blood clots further slowed the already retarded blood flow up from his leg veins.

6. After the removal of the pelvic blood clots, he developed additional clotting of the stagnant blood inside his leg veins, resulting in marked swelling (edema) of his legs.

In summary: a postnatal irritation and blockage of the vena cava; a posttraumatic, intra-abdominal hemorrhage; and a postoperative thrombophlebitis. *Diagnosis clinched!* (Mark your score cards "London to Gaynor to Levine.")

Little Michael's blocked vena cava was a time bomb, detonated 27 years later by the right fist of his nephew. Michael is now 31 and enjoying good, uninteresting health with the exception of his mildly swollen legs for which he will take anticoagulant therapy the rest of his life.

Michael's interesting case has several ramifications of importance to patients and physicians in this age of Managed Care. First is the immense value of pooling medical brain power when an "interesting case" is threatening to become a fatal one. The late, great Dr. Levine, hematologist extraordinaire, asked the key question that lifted the final veil from Michael's maddeningly elusive diagnosis. Under managed care, you will never find the likes of a Dr. Levine.

Michael's condition was unique in my experience, but not in Dr. Levine's. Every doctor I've talked to has encountered a case or two of an illness, the likes of which are rarely, if ever, described in medical textbooks or journals. A unique illness is not rare. Some, like Michael's, are caused by physicians—"iatrogenic illnesses." (Rather than say "physician-caused diseases," we prefer to use a term that's Greek to most people.)

Patients are well advised to eat prudently, exercise, be born without complications, have health insurance that provides easy access to specialists, and be aware that it's safer to give therapy than to receive it.

Each night I pray that I may never see another interesting case—or become one myself.

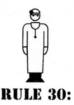

RULE 30:

May You Never Have to Give "The Look"

In more than 30 years of medical practice, I've seen The Look just three times. I pray that I never see it again. The Look is the expression on the face of patients who not only fear they are about to die, but who *know* they are about to die. As a doctor, I can provide reassurance to those who just think they are dying; often they are merely having a panic attack from which they will fully recover. But on each of the three occasions when I was the object of The Look, I was at a complete loss to know what to do for the patients, since I agreed with them—they were about to die. Within a half-hour of giving me The Look, each one did.

The first patient was Ingrid, a beautiful, 21-year-old Norwegian secretary, recently married to Rick, a handsome American executive in his early thirties. He had met her in Oslo on a business trip. He told me later that the moment she looked up at him from her desk and smiled, he fell in love with her. That look was the exact opposite of the one she gave me just before she died.

During their engagement, she told him that she had suffered from diabetes since childhood, but that it appeared to be well-controlled on insulin. They spent their honeymoon in a Paris hospital where she was successfully treated for diabetic coma. Lab tests in Paris established that she suffered from severe diabetic kidney disease. The young couple was thunderstruck. Since being started on insulin at the age of 10, she had not felt ill for 11 years. Despairing, they returned from their honeymoon in France to their new home in Northern California.

I first met her in 1960 when I was a medical resident on the renal service at Stanford Medical Center. She died under my care, almost a year later. This was just before the advent of the artificial kidney and renal transplant surgery, miracles of technology that have since revolutionized the treatment of chronic kidney disease.

Having been assigned to care for this young patient, I first met her and her husband in the outpatient department. To this day, I've never crossed paths with a more splendid looking married couple more hopelessly in love. Kidney disease is a silent killer and until I looked at her laboratory tests, I could not have imagined that this vibrant woman had less than a year to live, or that she and her husband had less than a year to love.

I worked in conjunction with a brilliant professor of nephrology to keep her feeling as good as possible for as long as possible. In those days, our relatively primitive weapons against renal disease included medications to control high blood pressure caused by kidney failure and nutritional advice about lowering the salt and protein content of the diet. I also strove for pinpoint control of her diabetes in order to slow down further damage to her kidneys. Most important, I served as a beacon of hope to them, a beacon that may have blinded them to the truth at the very end of her life.

They always arrived for her visit to the renal clinic impeccably dressed and holding hands. They always left arm in arm. It was immediately apparent to me that I was not treating one patient, but two. She and her husband hung on every one of the few hopeful words I was able to offer. The professor was able to provide them only with the comfort of his prestige.

They insisted on being told the truth about her condition and before long, they could interpret her gradually worsening laboratory values as well as any doctor. "How's my creatinine this week?" became her routine opening remark, always with an expectant smile. Ingrid laughed and cried easily and spoke with a slight Norwegian accent, punctuated by frequent little gasps of comprehension, which only made me more irretrievably attracted to her and her plight, and her husband's.

As the year wore on, she gradually weakened and her face became slightly puffy. Eventually, it was necessary to restrict her intake of fluid. Her appetite vanished.

One afternoon, while I was checking her blood pressure, Ingrid suddenly screamed and grasped her head in her hands. Her husband jumped to her side and hugged her. I stepped back in time to receive The Look over her husband's shoulder. She had just suffered a brain hemorrhage that would kill her in a few minutes. This diagnosis was clear to me the moment she reached for her head. Her husband and I helped her lie down on the examining table. I asked that he run to the nurse's station to bring help. For the last time, I took her blood pressure: extremely high at 280 over 140, the result this time of brain hemorrhage rather than kidney disease.

In the past, she was always eager to ask me about her blood-pressure reading. This time she gave me The Look. Helplessly, I clutched her shoulder above the blood-pressure cuff, squeezed hard and looked into her terrified blue eyes. Her dilated pupils were a shiny black. Her pale skin was cold in my grip. Instinctively, I was trying to give her a transfusion of my strength as hers rapidly waned. By the time the professor, other doctors, nurses, and her husband rushed into the room, her pupils were still dilated, not from fear, but from death. The luster was gone.

I didn't see The Look again for another 10 years, by which time I was in the private practice of internal medicine. On this occasion, it was another beautiful woman who gave me The Look. Linda was in her mid-30s and at the height of her career as a molecular biologist. What was remarkable about her, besides her uncanny resemblance to Ava Gardner, was that she had risen so far in the intellectually demanding field of molecular biology on only a high school education. Through the years, a succession of acclaimed male biologists had been drawn to her, first by her beauty and ultimately by her shining intelligence. In less than five years, she worked her way up from a lab assistant who washed glassware to a major contributor of landmark medical research.

When she first told me the story of her career, I felt resentment at the teachers who failed to recognize her awesome intelligence and creativity during her impoverished childhood. Fifteen years after she graduated high school, her name began appearing on a number of important scientific papers, but because of her humble educational background, she was listed far below other researchers who had lofty credentials and half her talent. Some of her work has led to therapies that have already saved thousands of lives. She died of a disease, sarcoma of the uterus, whose treatment still remains primitive and punishing.

A divorced, working mother of a 10-year-old boy, she first consulted me because of increasing fatigue during the previous year. When she recited her schedule—seven 12-hour days a week at the lab, four hours daily with her son, two hours of housework, five hours of sleep—I thought I didn't have to look farther for an explanation of her fatigue. I was wrong. Her initial lab tests showed she was severely anemic. Worse, her physical exam revealed a huge mass in her uterus and an enlarged liver. I shared her forlorn, tearful hope that she had sought medical advice in time to cure her.

I referred her to a gynecologist who soon removed her cancer-swollen uterus, but not before the tumor had spread to her liver, a sarcoma being one of the fastest growing of all cancers. She was begun on chemotherapy which seemed to arrest further spread for a while, at the cost of her lovely brown hair and months of nausea and vomiting. After trying to work part-time at the lab, she again appeared at my office, this time complaining of double vision. Her exam showed unmistakable evidence that the tumor had spread to her brain.

By now, she had lost 20 pounds from a beautifully proportioned figure that had always been lean. With her hairless scalp and frail body, she resembled an inmate of Auschwitz; I have since looked on cancer as a Nazi.

She was not one to be comforted by half-truths. I told her that she would have to see a neurosurgeon in hopes that brain surgery might give her temporary respite from her brain tumor. When she heard this, she gave me a level, brown-eyed gaze and said, "Thank you."

She gave me The Look a week later, when she was about to be wheeled into the operating room for a desperate neurosurgical attempt to add a few months to her life or, as she saw it, add a few months of motherhood to her son's life. At first, Linda glanced up from her gurney and joked that she was doubly comforted at seeing two of me. I was too upset to smile back. The next moment, the orderly gave the gurney an initial push and she gave me The Look.

Once again at a loss, I clasped her right hand firmly and stared back at her. This time the irises I gazed down at were brown, but the pupils were huge, black, and glittering. As she was wheeled down the hall, I walked alongside, squeezing her ice-cold hand with my slightly warmer one. She squeezed back. Just before she glided into the sterile confines of the operating room and the oblivion of anesthesia, her hand went limp in mine. Her life ran out like water between my fingers. She was wheeled dead to the operating table and was not able to be resuscitated.

The last time I saw The Look was five years ago when Gary, a 54-year-old African-American, who had just retired from the Police Department after 30 years, was writhing in chest pain from a heart attack. The night before, he had dined with his family at an excellent restaurant where he enjoyed his last meal and his last cigarette before doubling up in pain.

He was admitted to the coronary care unit of our local hospital where his EKG showed evidence of ischemia: an inadequate oxygen supply to his heart muscle. A routine chest X-ray taken at the bedside revealed a small cancer in his left lower lung.

I had been urging him to quit smoking for 20 years. All I received for my efforts were his charming smile and a dismissive shake of his head. I always thought he looked like a deeply tanned Douglas Fairbanks, Jr., complete with dapper mustache and devil-may-care grin.

Shortly after I admitted him to the C.C.U., he touched the plastic oxygen tube clipped to his nostrils and gave me his Fairbanks smile. "I never thought it would be so easy to quit smoking," he said. "All it took was a heart attack and cancer."

Despite huge doses of intravenous morphine, his chest pain persisted. In the middle of the night, I asked a cardiac surgeon to see him. The surgeon proposed a dramatic maneuver to save Gary's life. He recommended not only doing a coronary bypass operation, but a resection of the lung cancer at the same time. "As long as we're in there, why not go for the whole enchilada?"

"Because," I said, "he'll almost certainly die during such a long procedure."

"Not in my operating room."

I suppose an overweening self-confidence is the first requirement of a successful surgeon, just as self-doubt may be the internist's greatest asset. After much thought, I advised the patient and his family to let the surgeon work on both his heart and lung. Gary was in too much pain and the family too stricken to object. By this time, he was in the agony of accelerated angina unresponsive to massive doses of narcotics. It took about 45 minutes for the surgeon to assemble his team and prepare the operating room.

While one of the surgical nurses was gently shaving the patient's chest, Gary grimaced in pain, then gave me The Look. It was the first humorless expression he had ever directed at me. Once again, all I could think to do was grip his arm tightly and stare back. I also turned up his morphine drip, to no avail. I wished that the president of the company that manufactured his favorite brand of cigarette were at the bedside to receive The Look instead of me.

A half hour into his operation, his heart stopped for the first time; ten minutes later, it stopped for the fifth and last time. When I told the family what happened, his wife said something I remember as vividly as The Look: "Well, thank God he didn't die of the cancer."

So far, I have been devastated by The Look three times. I'm never prepared for it. The Look not only expresses the ultimate horror, but also signals the patient's feeling of betrayal by his suddenly helpless doctor. The Look is more than I can bear. "Do something!" it screams. All I can do is grab the patient for dear life and glare back in a futile effort to stare down The Look. I'm not going to insult someone at the very end of life by returning The Look with The Lie: "Everything's going to be fine."

How can you under Managed Care forestall having to give your doctor The Look? Actually, through its emphasis on prevention, Managed Care might well help you defer your final moment for years.

If you've had diabetes since childhood, as the first patient did, you could do worse than finding an internist who will help you tightly control your blood sugars with as many as four daily insulin injections, each followed by a feeding. Pinpoint diabetic control is the best prevention of the disastrous consequences of this disease, including what led to this patient's death—end-stage renal disease with secondary hypertension culminating in a brain hemorrhage.

Nowadays, kidney transplants are available under Managed Care to young patients with end-stage renal disease. Whether Managed Care similarly covers older patients remains to be seen. Peruse your health insurance policy. I don't think Managed Care, let alone the patient, should be stuck with the huge bill for renal dialysis or a kidney transplant; end-stage renal disease is one of those medical catastrophes the government should cover.

If your diabetes has been discovered during adulthood, chances are you're overweight. You might spare your doctor The Look by joining one of the weight reduction programs sponsored by Managed Care.

The second patient, who died of uterine cancer, sends an urgent preventive message that Managed Care endorses: Get an annual pelvic exam and Pap smear. These routine, boring medical rituals are your best hope of preventing an exciting medical crisis such as emergency surgery for massive hemorrhage from uterine cancer. What you don't want to be is an exciting case.

The third patient, who suffered from lung cancer and fatal heart disease, might still be alive today if he had access to one of the successful smoking cessation programs now sponsored by Managed Care.

Under fee-for-service, I was not able to prevent these three patients from giving me The Look. Would they have done better under Managed Care? I doubt it, but who knows? Don't look at me.

RULE 31:

A Safe Bet on the Four Horsemen of the Apocalypse Is War to Show, Pestilence to Place, and Death to Win

Under Managed Care, we doctors are encouraged to practice pre-emptive, rather than reactive, medicine—boring preventive medicine, rather than exciting, blood and guts medicine. Perhaps a knowledge of what is most likely to kill you at a given age might stimulate you to take the necessary, boring measures to stick around a bit longer.

It's too bad 50 years have to pass before we get religion about our own health. It's either pure luck or our parents' vigilance that gets us through ages one to four when the major cause of death is drowning, or ages 19 to 39 when the leading causes (in order) are motor vehicle accidents, homicide, suicide, other injuries, and heart disease. Young adults are the lost generation of preventive medicine; they see their doctors only for acute illnesses. If young patients see me for a sprained thumb, they can't leave my office until I've inflicted on them my hellfire and brimstone lecture on booze, cigarettes, condoms, seat belts, firearms, and bicycle helmets. Sometimes I think that all I succeed in doing to these kids is instilling in them a fierce desire to protect their thumbs from re-injury so they never have to see me again.

Between ages 40 and 64 we're zapped by heart disease, lung cancer, stroke, breast cancer, colorectal cancer, and chronic lung disease. By this time of life, the dairy and tobacco industries have milked us dry and smoked us out. They turn their attention over our dead bodies to the teenage market with its virginal lungs and pristine blood vessels.

At age 65, we see the final posting of the odds for the running of the last mile. A wreath of roses awaits us at the finish line. The field of six breaks down as follows: Heart Disease (by Cholesterol, out of Nicotine), Stroke (by Cholesterol, out of Hypertension), Chronic Lung Disease (by Phillip Morris, out of Virginia Slims), Pneumonia (by Strep, out of Nursing Home), Lung Cancer (by Marlboro, out of Lucky Strike), and Colorectal Cancer (by Obesity, out of Heredity). And they're off!

God knows we're beautifully set up in this country to react to lung cancer with surgery, radiation, and chemotherapy. This represents a million-dollar treatment for a two-dollar disease, the cost of your first pack of cigarettes. Our medical personnel are superbly trained, the equipment is high-tech and gleaming, and if anyone can give you the best odds on beating lung cancer—5 percent survival after five years—it's that great handicapper, the American doctor.

On the other hand, the preemptive solution to lung cancer is much less dramatic and much more difficult. It requires giving up cigarettes, a $400 treatment that includes a visit to your doctor, a full six-week course of nicotine patches, and group counseling. You can readily see why Managed Care would rather pay for this type of treatment for lung cancer than the million-dollar alternative. On the other hand, removing a malignant nodule from a lung is a lot easier than removing a cigarette from a mouth because during the first procedure, the patient is asleep.

I'm forever amazed that when I routinely ask patients if they smoke, the answer is frequently a sheepish "Yes," and from the most unlikely people—offspring of lung cancer patients, college professors, pulmonary therapists, asthmatics, pregnant women, and mothers of infant children. I'm even more amazed to learn that most doctors fail to ask their patients if they smoke.

About the only other disease with a worse cure rate than lung cancer is obesity—just 2 percent of successful dieters stay lean after five years. Nutrition is one of the soupiest of medical sciences and too many cooks are spoiling the broth. Out of all the conflicting advice you get from these nutritionists, two facts emerge: if you want to be vigorous in your 80s, you have to eat much less fat and lots more vegetables; and, if you're one of the 50 percent of Americans who are overweight, it's fairly easy to lose weight and almost impossible to keep it off. You be an exception, as I am.

Finally, you mustn't forget to exercise. If you take a cruise aboard the Love Boat, be sure to put in at least a half hour a day on the rowing machine in the fitness center. It took mankind 4000 years to evolve from a galley slave to a passenger on a cruise ship, and it appears to me as I gaze into the fitness center that we're backsliding.

A rather vigorous weight-lifting program has recently been shown to help nursing home patients feel better, fall less often, and live longer. Oh terrific! We come to the end of life in a rest home when all we want is a little rest, then some Brunhilde wakes us up each morning at six to lift weights. Oy. You really want to feel better? Stay in bed and listen to your fellow inmates grunting down the hall in the weight room. Be careful you don't laugh so hard you fall out of bed.

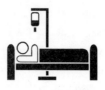

RULE 32:

At the End of Your Life, Ask Your Doctor to Help You Out

It's not uncommon for doctors (including this one) to prescribe a morphine drip for a dying patient who is suffering intense pain. A doctor is grateful to any patient who signs a durable power of attorney for health care so that the family or a friend can participate with the doctor and patient in this decision to relieve the pain. The morphine undoubtedly hastens the inevitable death, but the patient dies in a state of mind approaching ecstasy, which is a marvelous parting gift from his or her loved ones.

In thinking about my own death, I would like to have a doctor care for me who will drip morphine into me in my final hours, not only if I'm suffering severe pain, but also if I'm merely suffering. An awareness of impending death is often a horrific experience, as I indicate in the chapter on The Look. If I give my doctor The Look, I'd like him or her to alter intravenously the expression on my face from horror to serenity.

Now comes the really controversial part. I hope that if I develop Alzheimer's disease and therefore lose all capacity to think straight, or remember what happened during the previous few minutes, or know who I am, I can be helped out of this life by morphine before I become both pathetic and an intolerable burden to my family.

Patients with Alzheimer's are blissfully pain-free themselves but unspeakably painful to their immediate family, as well as a bottomless pit of expense. The possibility of inflicting this pain on my own family in the future is extremely painful to me now. I look on this mental anguish as a bottled up emotion which I have now set adrift in the downstream of time. The doctor who retrieves my bottle will read this message:

Dear Doctor,

If you and a qualified neurologist determine that I am irreversibly demented, with virtually no awareness of time, place, or recent events, I request that you consider my body a permanent reservoir of the intense pain I feel as I write this. This severe pain of mine is over the suffering my illness will be causing my family by the time you read this. Although I will likely deny being in pain when I am demented, please be assured that the pain is still within me and I implore you, through means of a morphine drip, to relieve it. With undying gratitude, I am,

Sincerely yours,
Oscar London, M.D.

I must be demented already to think I'd ever find a doctor to do me and my family this kindness.

RULE 33:

Never Take the Stairs when You Can Take the Elevator

Thanks to the hatchet job Managed Care is doing on the American hospital, all that will be left standing inside this venerable institution by the year 2000 will be the lobby elevator. Behind its sliding doors will be crowded many poignant memories.

Lost in thought, I waited in the lobby of Alta Bates Hospital in Berkeley to take the elevator up to Four West, the Medical Unit. As the bronze doors slid open, an older colleague of mine, whom I hadn't seen for a year, materialized at my side and stepped into the elevator with me. "How've you been, Dave," I said, observing that he looked somewhat thinner than I remembered him. He nodded, and smiled weakly. "Fourth floor?" I asked. Before I could push the button, he reached in front of me and pressed "B," for the basement. Then I knew. He had terminal cancer. In the basement of Alta Bates resides the Radiation Therapy Department. Before the doors closed, I hopped back out into the lobby and called over my shoulder, "I'll catch the next one, Dave. Good luck." He nodded again, but did not smile as the doors sealed him, alone, inside the wood-paneled box, going down. I have never in my life seen a more desolate expression on anyone's face.

When the hospital elevators run a bit slowly, which is not a rare phenomenon, a small crowd gathers in the lobby, waiting for a lift. A diagnostician by trade, I often try to guess the destinations of my fellow travelers. The basement, as I mentioned, is all too easy, and ghastly, to figure out. The third floor is an equally simple destination to deduce, but, in contrast to the basement and in general direction, it is pure heaven. I don't have to ask the beaming young man, holding flowers in one hand and strings of large helium balloons in the other, what floor he wants. I automatically beam him up to Three, the Labor and Delivery Unit. Even a layman can figure out a third-floor destination when five married couples—the playful men holding pillows to their abdomens to mimic their pregnant wives—wait to ascend to their Lamaze class.

A more subtle discernment is required to diagnose the destinations of visitors to the Medical Unit (Four), the Surgical Unit (Five), and the Intensive Care Unit (I.C.U., Six). Visitors bound for Four will confront languishing patients who are too sick to go home and not sick enough to qualify for the I.C.U. on Six. As a result of their slow recovery from such maladies as strokes, pneumonias, and phlebitis, patients on Four attract a chronically pensive and terminally bored set of visitors. Their gifts, if any, are devoid of the levity of helium balloons or even the wickedness of chocolate. The limply beribboned, rectangular boxes in their arthritic hands contain, I surmise, pink bed jackets for the female patients and brown slippers for the male. Or the melancholy visitors to Four might bear a few chemically burned, home-grown blossoms whose frail stems cling to life-support in a wad of moist Kleenex. In my opinion, a fourth-floor patient receiving these reminders of neglected gardening chores has a disincentive to recover.

In general—I am a generalist by profession—visitors to surgical patients on Five seem to be somewhat younger and happier, and bring more upbeat offerings. For example, a green-glazed Japanese pot containing a spray of white, scarlet-centered orchids. To my trained and slightly crazed eye, the orchids resemble a row of gauze sponges lightly bloodied by a softly whistling surgeon closing an appendectomy wound. "Fifth floor?" I confidently ask, and the surgical visitors and their bloody orchids nod in unison.

The vast majority of surgical patients survive their operations and anesthetics to enjoy, with their visitors, a steady recovery. By contrast, there are the inoperable patients who are sequestered in what amounts to a cancer ward in a remote wing of the fourth floor. Their visitors have a haunted look, their tragic eyes long ago drained of anxiety and tears.

The eyes also announce the destination of visitors to the I.C.U. These are the terrified eyes of those fearful of losing a loved one. With pupils dilated, their eyes glitter with apprehension as they wait to be lifted from lobby to sixth floor. If their worst fears are realized, they will hide their tear-streaming eyes behind handkerchiefs during their descent from Intensive Care to indifferent lobby.

The elevators are also a means of studying physicians while they are between patients and floors. A doctor in an elevator—a doc in a box—is a fish out of water. Doctors are most comfortable confronting other human beings within the autocracy of the office or hospital room. In the democracy of an elevator, they rise and fall in tandem with everyone else and can't wait to disembark.

To stand out from the crowd and not, God forbid, be mistaken for a civilian, doctors employ various sartorial strategies. In vain. The long, white coat, alas, no longer identifies just a doctor, but also a nursing supervisor, lab technician, or, as I noted the other day, a delivery boy for a florist. I have taken to wearing a navy-blue blazer and light-gray flannel slacks, which happen to be the uniform of the plainclothes security guards as well as that of male hospital administrators (who, these days, seem to outnumber the patients and doctors combined). To distinguish myself from members of these honorable professions, I have variously tried wearing my hospital-issue, plastic name tag (tacky) or my stethoscope (ostentatious). My beeper could as easily signify a well-heeled drug dealer as a down-at-the-heels internist. What ultimately distinguishes me from the imperious administrator, the affluent cocaine courier, and the furtive security guard is the hangdog expression I uniformly wear on my face—the visage of an internist in the age of Managed Care. "Pretty rough, ain't it, Doc?" is a greeting I'm often given from perfect strangers in the hospital elevator.

Before they were instructed not to, surgeons used to swagger onto elevators and through hospital corridors in their skimpy, green scrub suits. These less than shy and far from retiring heroes were the Schwarzennegers, Seagals, and Stallones of surgery—no mistaking *them* in their rumpled, green battle fatigues. Under the current hospital dress code, surgeons are required to cover up. As a result, they've taken to wearing their tweed sports jackets on top of their turtle-green scrub pants—a sartorial disaster second only to the visiting-team attire of the Toronto Bluejays.

Non-surgical, female physicians have a more daunting identity problem. Dressed in smart, tailored suits, they not only resemble female hospital administrators, they can easily be mistaken for social workers, yuppie visitors, or, heaven forfend, drug-company representatives. Eschewing stethoscopes and name tags, as I have, the female physician is too dignified to permit her face to fall into the natural hangdog look of an internist, or be stretched into the gung ho, can-do smile of a surgeon. Instead, she chooses to wear no makeup, and to assume the serene expression of a self-sacrificing professional who has made it in what, a scant ten years ago, was a man's world. I, for one, have no trouble spotting a new female colleague. She's the one who smiles at me collegially and sympathetically.

One of the more touching scenes I've encountered inside the hospital elevator is the doctor making rounds with his or her child on a weekend. Here's a 38-year-old, fiercely mustached orthopedic surgeon holding the hand of his four-year-old son, who looks up at his dad and asks, "Can I push Five?" At four years, the son already knows where his dad works, but, more important, the dad is bonding with his son. And most important, he's letting his wife, the obstetrician, sleep in on Saturday morning.

Yesterday, while waiting for the elevator, I saw, walking slowly toward me, one of my least favorite patients, a whiney gentleman in his late 80s whose endless complaints had already taken 10 years off my life. "Oh, no!" I thought. Since he had not yet noticed me, I turned my back to him and thought of bolting down the long lobby to the elevator in the south wing. Suddenly, I remembered that the patient I had in mind had died three years ago. The gentleman limping toward me merely resembled him!

Filled with a combination of guilt at snubbing a patient after he'd died and anxiety over my failing powers of observation and memory, I impatiently pressed the elevator button for the third time. The doors suddenly swung open to reveal my favorite sight in medicine: a first-time mother in a balloon-festooned wheelchair, cradling her sleeping newborn in her arms. Looking as happy and haggard as his wife, the first-time father tenderly pushed the wheelchair out of the elevator and into the lobby. Two sets of grandparents and a nurse's aid brought up the rear. I stared in awe and delight, conjecturing that if that baby girl ever grew up to become the Rose Bowl Queen or the President, her float or motorcade could never approach in grandeur this slow, homeward-bound procession through the lobby of Alta Bates Hospital.

Ever since my appendectomy at age 15, I've missed the little guy. Don't ask me why I've longed for this severed, vestigal organ; it's simply a gut feeling of mine. Much as some people spend their adulthood in a quest for their long-lost father, I have been searching for my missing little worm. I am very pleased to announce that after more than 40 years, I finally came across it at the very end of this book.

APPENDIX:

You Can't Survive Managed Care without Your Personal Health Guide

Y our HMO, in its private memos, does not refer to you as "patients" or even "people." It calls you "lives," as in "we've signed up 3000 more lives this year than last." If your HMO has not had to fork out too much on your dying, it looks with sorrow on your death as the brutal curtailment of premium payments. Managed care regrets that you have but one life to give to your HMO.

Under Managed Care, my overworked staff and I are too busy to remind you that it's high time I recheck your blood pressure. We can hardly spare the time to satisfy your curiosity about how low your LDL cholesterol was last year or to tell you when you had your last tetanus shot. In the spirit of managing your own care, you should have this data at your fingertips.

I urge you to send away for a small, 3 X 5-inch, 32-page booklet called *Put Prevention into Practice—Personal Health Guide.* Published by the U.S. Department of Health and Human Services, it may save your life. It's the civilian equivalent of the small, bulletproof Bible soldiers used to slip into their breast pockets before going into battle. After studying your *Personal Health Guide,* carry it in a pocket over your heart and it may stop a bullet-sized blood clot from lodging in your left main coronary artery. (Obtain copies of the *Personal Health Guide* by writing Consumer Information Center, Pueblo, CO 81009. Copies cost $1.00 each. Specify item 151A and quantity. Make checks payable to Superintendent of Documents.)

Bring it along with you every time you see your doctor. With a few well-placed notes, the two of you can compose your own health Bible, writing such commandments as: "Mammograms each year in February; cholesterol check every April and November; pneumonia shot at 65; 20-pound weight loss by May 1; no cigarettes after March 3, 1996."

Doctors' notes are imperfect at best. Your help is needed. With this succinct, well-organized booklet, you can instantly retrieve records of your blood pressure, cholesterol values, immunizations, original weight before dieting, and date of last Pap smear, in your own legible handwriting.

At the same time, your *Personal Health Guide* will remind you of such things as the importance of no-slip rugs and smoke alarms, give you dietary guidelines and instruct you to keep the temperature of your home's hot water at less than 120°F. You can look on your *Personal Health Guide* as an owner's manual for your body. The more you ignore your manual, the sooner your lifetime warranty expires.

After all, Death keeps a ledger on you. In his little black book embossed with your name, Death records such things as how many cigarettes you smoke, how much extra weight you haul, how many millimeters above normal your blood pressure reads, how often you fail to wear your seat belt, how fast you drive on the freeway, how many hours you sit before the boob tube, and how many ounces of gin you drink each day. When these deadly stats add up to three score and ten, no matter what your chronological age, Death, with a smile, can close his book on you.

In contrast to that little black book, your *Personal Health Guide* is a book of life. Until you get your copy, here's its list of mostly toll-free numbers through which you can get the lowdown from high-ups on how to live better and longer.

Aging

National Council on Aging
(800) 424-9046

AIDS

CDC National AIDS Hotline
(800) 342-AIDS

Alcohol and Drug Abuse

National Clearing House for Alcohol and Drug Information
(800) 729-6686

Cancer

Cancer Information Service
(800) 4-CANCER

Child Abuse

National Child Abuse Hotline
(800) 422-4453

Food and Drug Safety

Food and Drug Administration, Office of Consumer Affairs
(301) 443-3170

Heart, Lung, and Blood Diseases

National Heart, Lung, and Blood Institute
Education Programs Center
(301) 951-3260

Maternal and Child Health

National Maternal and Child Health Clearinghouse
(703) 821-8955, Ext. 254

Mental Health

National Mental Health Association
(800) 969-6642

Occupational Safety and Health

National Institute for Occupational Safety and Health
(800) 356-4674

Physical Activity and Fitness

Aerobic and Fitness Foundation
(800) BE FIT 86

Safety and Injury Prevention

Consumer Product Safety Commission
(800) 638-CPSC

National Highway Traffic Safety Administration,
Auto Safety Hotline
(800) 424-9393

Sexually Transmitted Diseases

CDC National STD Hotline
(800) 227-8922

PUBLISHER'S NOTE: Oscar London, M.D., W.B.D. has asked us to inform you that he wishes you all the best under Managed Care. Having dared to reveal his darkest secrets of how to survive Managed Care, he has joined the Federal Internist Relocation Program. Aging gracefully somewhere in the continental United States, he is no longer available for consultation. Dr. Generic will see you now.